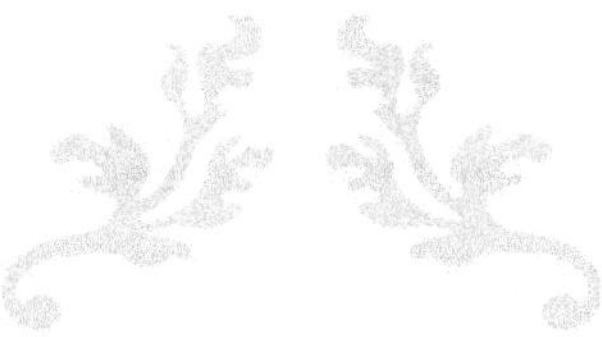

Raising Your Vibration

with Essential Oils

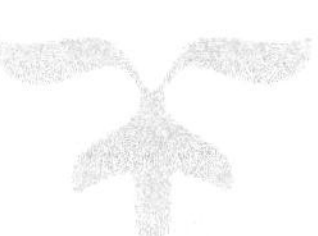

Copyright © 2023 *Mary Mauchly*

Table of Contents

Introduction

Holistic and alternative methods of improving one's health and well-being have gained popularity in recent years. The use of essential oils is one such strategy that, although having been around for thousands of years, is becoming more and more popular recently as people seek more holistic methods as they attempt to reduce their toxic load. These potent plant extracts have been used for ages in aromatherapy and conventional treatment. Essential oils are thought to have the power to affect and raise our vibrational frequency in addition to their affect physically, emotionally, and aromatically.

This idea, rooted in mysticism and ancient wisdom and quantum physics, contends that everything in the cosmos, including our mental, emotional, and spiritual states, vibrate at particular frequencies. It is thought that by utilising the power of essential oils, we can increase our vibrational frequency, improve our lives as we feel more harmony, balance, and energy. Here we will discuss the idea of vibrational frequency, the possible advantages of essential oils, and how to employ them to enhance our general well-being.

Learning About Vibrational Frequency

The pace at which an energy source or object vibrates is called vibrational frequency. Everything in the cosmos, including our ideas, emotions, and physical bodies, vibrates at a particular frequency, according to quantum physics and spiritual beliefs. We feel a sense of well-being, joy, and vigour when our vibrational frequency is in harmony with our desires and the natural flow of energy. On the other hand, imbalances, stress, and illness can result when our vibrational frequency is low or interrupted.

Essential Oils: A Guide to Their Qualities

Essential oils are extracts that are heavily concentrated and are obtained from different plant components, such as flowers, leaves, stems, and roots. These oils' distinctive scents and healing qualities result from the aromatic molecules they contain. Since every essential oil has a particular chemical makeup, it can be used for various things. While some are energising and invigorating, other oils are noted for their calming and relaxing properties. Some oils have anti-histamine, anti-viral, anti-bacterial, or anti-inflammatory qualities, increasing their potential health benefits.

Essential Oils and Vibrational Frequency Enhancement

The idea that essential oils have distinctive vibrational energy underlies their usage to raise the vibrational frequency. It is believed that when essential oils come into contact with us, whether through inhalation or topical application, their vibrational frequency interacts with our own, esentially affecting our energy field and general wellbeing. We can deliberately work towards increasing our vibrational frequency by choosing essential oils that resonate with our desired states.

Understanding that essential oils cannot significantly alter our vibrational frequency is vital. They should be utilised as a component of a comprehensive strategy that also incorporates personal development, healthy lifestyle choices, and mindfulness techniques. However, adding essential oils to our daily routine can be a potent tool for enhancing our vibrational frequency and supporting our general health.

Choosing Essential Oils to Improve Vibration

When choosing essential oils to raise the vibrational frequency, it is crucial to consider the purity of the oils. Standardized oils are generally adulterated with synthetic fragrences so that they can deliver a consistent smell from one product to the next. What this means is that they may include other elements like carrier oils or other synthetic components. With lack of governance on ingredient lables in the essential oil businesses world wide, there are no mandates on labeling as of yet. Take the time to research the company that produces the oils. What their growing and sourcing practices are, what their testing practices are, and do they contribute to sound environmental practices. When you consider that your skin is your bodys first line of defense, why would you use anything toxic or less than certified therapeutic grade?

Different oils are linked to particular energies and qualities that can complement various parts of our wellbeing. Lavender oil, for example, is well known for its relaxing and soothing properties, making it excellent for fostering balance and relaxation. Contrarily, citrus oils with uplifting and energising properties, such as lemon or grapefruit, boost mood and motivation.

Making blends or synergistic oil mixtures can also enhance individual oils' benefits. Blocking fats with complementary characteristics can create a harmonic and balanced fragrant experience that resonates with our desired state of vibration. Finding the blend of oils that works best for each person requires a lot of experimentation and intuition.

Approaches to Application

There are many ways to use essential oils to raise the vibrational frequency. One of the most efficient techniques is inhalation since the molecules of the oils are readily absorbed through the respiratory system and directly impact the limbic system, which regulates emotions and memory. A diffuser can be filled with a few drops of essential oil for inhalation, or the oil can be breathed directly from the bottle. Relaxation, mental clarity, and emotional equilibrium can all be benefited from this practise.

Topical usage is a different approach to application. Applying essential oils to the skin requires diluting them with carrier oils like coconut, almond, grapeseed or jojoba oil. The therapeutic benefits of essential oils and the physical advantages of touch are combined in the well-liked massage technique. Applying oils to particular body parts, such as the wrists, temples, or soles of the feet, enables simple absorption and fosters well-being all day long.

Using certain essential oils in a specific sequence and application allows one to address a specific body system and/or area of the body, providing a focused approach to the symptoms and underlying causes of many ailments and illnesses.

Essential oils can also be utilised in baths, showers, meditation, visualisation techniques, inhalation, and physical application. A warm bath can be made luxurious and scented by adding a few drops of essential oil, which can help the body and mind unwind. Alternately, inhaling the steam from a shower while dabbing a few drops of oil on a washcloth or sponge can energise and uplift the senses.

The Use of Essential Oils for Vibrational Frequency Has Many Advantages.

Using essential oils to raise vibrational frequency has a variety of possible advantages. As we increase our vibrational frequency, we could notice:

Increased Vitality and Energy: Some essential oils, like citrus or peppermint, are well known for their energising and uplifting qualities. These oils can help increase energy levels and improve general vitality when inhaled or applied topically during a massage.

Emotional Balance: Essential oils can affect how we feel and how we respond to situations. Calming oils like lavender or chamomile can facilitate relaxation and decrease tension and anxiety. Conversely, mood-lifting oils that encourage a positive approach include bergamot and ylang-ylang.

Spiritual Connection: Numerous essential oils have been used for years to improve contemplation, prayer, and meditation. Frankincense and sandalwood oils, for example, are thought to heighten spiritual awareness and develop a sense of oneness with Source.

Focus and Mental Clarity: Some essential oils, like Intune *, peppermint or rosemary, are renowned for stimulating and clearing the mind. Concentration, memory, and mental clarity can be improved by inhaling or utilising these oils during study or work.

Physical Well-Being: Essential oils' different therapeutic properties can promote physical wellness. For instance, lavender promotes relaxation but also is an antihistimine. Eucalyptus oil helps support respiratory health, while tea tree oil has antibacterial characteristics. Including these oils in a wellness regimen can improve general physical health.

Using essential oils to raise vibrational frequency is a holistic method that blends the power of aromatherapy, natural healing, and spirituality. Despite the low historical studies of vibrational frequency that has been in the layman's field of view, or of scientific studies on the specific effects of essential oils on vibrational frequency, many people have experienced exceptional outcomes and advantages from using essential oils regularly. It's critical to approach this practice with an open mind and an eagerness to investigate and identify the essential oils that speak to our needs and aspirations.

Never forget that essential oils should be considered an additional practice rather than a replacement for qualified medical or psychiatric care. Always seek advice from a healthcare professional before using essential oils if you have any underlying medical ailments or concerns. We may improve our health, foster balance, and elevate our vibratory frequency to live a more peaceful and contented existence by embracing the possibilities of essential oils and incorporating them into a comprehensive self-care routine. There are holistic healthcare professionals that have studied the "old world" remedies, and seek to provide care that supports your body's natural ability to heal itself. I include in my recommendations for a holistic approach to healthy and high vibe living the use of accupuncture, homeopathy, chiropractic, cranio sacral and massage therapies along with Reiki and essential oils.

Chapter 1: Energy underlies everything!

Since ancient times, people of all nations and spiritual systems have accepted that the universe is entirely of energy. This idea is based on the conviction that all matter, including intangible components like thoughts and emotions, is composed of vibrating energy. According to quantum physics, power exists in all shapes and frequencies and constantly interacts with and affects the environment.

This viewpoint contends that individuals have distinctive energetic vibrations due to being a part of the vast, interconnected web of energy. Our ideas, feelings, physical bodies, and surroundings produce and absorb energy. We feel well-being, vibrancy, and alignment with the world when our energy is balanced and in accord and we experience positive coincidences in our lives. On the other hand, when our energy is disturbed or unbalanced, it can result in discord in our bodily, emotional, and spiritual selves, and we experience a series of unfortunate events that we cannot understand 'why this always happens to me'.

With their concentrated and strong qualities, essential oils have long been recognised as instruments for influencing and harnessing energy. These oils, made from various plant components, including flowers, leaves, stems, and roots, contain the spirit and life energy of the source material. The energy vibrations of the plants from which essential oils are collected are said to be carried by them.

The energetic characteristics of essential oils are supposed to alter our energy field when we engage with them by affecting our emotions, which is the biggest contributor to your vibrational output. Whether through inhalation, topical application, or ingestion (with caution and with the help of a qualified professional), with their distinct vibrational frequencies, we can intentionally engage with essential oils to balance, enhance, and transform our energetic states.

Since ancient times, essential oils have been employed in various healing practices, currency, conventional medical procedures, including aromatherapy, Ayurveda, and Chinese medicine. They have also been incorporated into spiritual and energy practices to promote rituals, energetic cleansing, and meditation. Every essential oil has unique active capabilities, and each can be chosen and used according to its these characteristics and intended use.

People aspire to harness the transforming power of essential oils to improve their emotions, and spiritual connection by incorporating them into their daily lives. They also utilise essential oils to balance their energy, enhance their vibrational frequency and advance general well-being.

In the following parts, we will delve into the energetic qualities of essential oils, discuss several methods for employing essential oils to improve and harness energy, and further explore the idea of energy and vibrational frequency. It is significant to note that, despite widespread use and anecdotal evidence, scientific research on the direct effects of essential oils on human energy and vibrational frequency is scarce. Therefore, it is crucial to approach the study of essential oils as tools for energy augmentation with an open mind, personal intuition, and a readiness to practise self-exploration and self-care.

Knowledge of essential oils

Numerous botanical sources' volatile chemicals and aromatic essences are captured in essential oils and highly concentrated plant extracts. They are known as "essential" because the plants from which they are derived are thought to contain their essence or life energy in them. Typically, essential oils are derived from various plant parts, including flowers, leaves, stems, bark, and roots.

The complicated chemical makeup of essential oils varies based on the type of plant used for extraction and its species. These include terpenes, esters, aldehydes, phenols, and ketones, among other chemical components. These substances help give essential oils their scent, medicinal effects, and prospective health advantages.

Essential oil sources and techniques of extraction

There are multiple ways to extract essential oils from plants, and each one is appropriate for specific plant types and intended results. Here are a few popular extraction techniques:

The most typical technique for obtaining essential oils is steam distillation. The plant material is heated with steam, which causes the volatile chemicals to evaporate. Following the condensation of the steam, an essential oil and water mixture is produced, which is then separated via a procedure known as decantation.

Citrus fruit essential oils are commonly extracted using the cold-pressing/expression technique. The essential oil is physically pressed out of the fruit's outer peel. The oil retains its original scent and medicinal qualities since no heat is involved in the cold pressing process.

For delicate flowers or plant materials that cannot tolerate the high temperatures of steam distillation, solvent extraction is used. The essential oil from the plant material is dissolved using a solvent, such as hexane or ethanol. The solvent is then expelled, leaving the essential oil behind.

Pressurised carbon dioxide is used in the CO2 extraction technique to extract essential oils. The aromatic components from the plant material are successfully extracted using CO2 as a solvent. Essential oils of the highest calibre and with a diverse spectrum of features are frequently produced through CO2 extraction.

Essential oils can be obtained from a wide variety of sources. They can be made from a variety of plant parts, including flowers (rose, lavender, for example), leaves (peppermint, eucalyptus), bark (cinnamon, cedarwood), roots (ginger, vetiver), resins (frankincense, myrrh), and many others. Each plant source has a distinct scent, medicinal benefits, and energetic qualities.

The essential oils' strength and concentration

Essential oils are potent and concentrated compounds. A lot of plant material is required to make a tiny amount of essential oil. For instance, it can require hundreds or even thousands of rose petals to produce just one drop of the oil. Essential oils' power and effectiveness come from their concentrated composition.

Essential oils should be used carefully and diluted appropriately due to their strength. Before being used on the skin or ear applications, they are often diluted with carrier oils like coconut or. Dilution not only increases absorption and lowers the chance of skin irritation, but it also ensures safety.

Because essential oils are very concentrated, a little goes a long way. Most essential oils only require a few drops for their fragrant and medicinal effects. It's crucial to respect the strength of essential oils, utilise them carefully, and follow the right instructions and suggestions.

The effectiveness of essential oils goes beyond only their physical attributes. They are valuable tools in energy work and holistic healing techniques since they are thought to carry the plants'nts' energetic vibrations and life f. People can access the energetic qualities of essential oils and their capacity to affect our energy states because of their concentrated nature.

Due to their concentrated nature, essential oils can influence our sensations and emotions. The limbic system, which is in charge of emotions and memory, is directly impacted by inhaling an essential oil's aroma through the olfactory system. Because of their proximity to the brain, essential oils can trigger strong emotional reactions and impact our mood and energy.

Additionally, essential oils are helpful for topical application due to their strength. The therapeutic characteristics of the oils can be distributed throughout the body when applied to the skin because they are absorbed and can enter the bloodstream. The oils can target particular locations, such as acupressure points or energy meridians, with this type of administration, giving our energetic system a more focused and localised effect.

Essential oils have a long shelf life due to their concentrated composition. Essential oils can last for a long time if appropriately stored due to the high concentration of volatile components in them. Therefore, They can be used easily and consistently to capture the energy and include them in routine self-care routines.

It's important to understand, though, that the strength of essential oils also calls for careful, informed application. Undiluted usage of some essential oils may irritate the skin, and some oils may need to be avoided by some people, such as those who are pregnant or have certain medical conditions. To ensure the correct and safe use of essential oils, it is imperative to seek the advice of trustworthy authorities like licenced aromatherapists or trustworthy reference materials.

Essential oils are extracts from various plant parts that have been greatly condensed. They have intricate volatile component mixtures contributing to their scent, medicinal qualities, and potential energising benefits. Due to their power, essential oils can significantly impact our overall health—physically, emotionally, and energetically. People can safely and intentionally use essential oils to enhance and harmonise their energetic states, fostering balance, vigour, and overall wellness. This is done by understanding the composition and concentrated nature of essential oils.

How vibrational frequency and energy affect our health

Our general health and well-being are significantly influenced by energy and vibrational frequency. The human body is more than just a physical structure; it is also an energetic system that communicates with and reacts to the energy in our environment. The following are some significant ways that energy and vibrational frequency affect human health:

Energetic harmony: We feel well-being, vitality, and peak performance when our body's energy is balanced and harmonious. Our active system's imbalances or blockages might appear as physical, emotional, or spiritual illnesses.

Emotional and Mental States: Our ideas, feelings, and mental states have vibrational frequency and energy. While negative emotions like fear, wrath, and despair are linked to lower frequencies, positive emotions like love, joy, and appreciation are linked to higher frequencies. The vibrational frequency of our emotional and mental states can impact our total energy and well-being. By consciously cultivating positive emotions and thoughts, we may increase our vibratory frequency and foster a better sense of positivity, resilience, and mental clarity.

Energetic Resonance: According to energetic resonance, things, substances, and even individuals with comparable vibrational frequencies are attracted and can impact one another. We may feel a good elevation in our energy when we are in places or surrounded by individuals who have higher vibrational frequencies. Negative or discordant energies, on the other hand, can be depleting to our well-being. Knowing the importance of vibrational frequency enables us to purposefully select settings and connections that promote our energetic resonance and general well-being.

Energetic Healing: Several holistic healing techniques, including Reiki, acupuncture, and sound therapy, is based on balancing and re-establishing the body's energetic flow. These techniques seek to clear energetic blockages, balance the body's vibrational frequency, and advance physical, emotional, and spiritual healing.

Conscious Intention and Manifestation: We can materialise our desires and objectives by raising our vibratory frequency through our thoughts, feelings, and intentions. Positive events, chances, and connections can enter our lives if our thoughts and aspirations are in tune with higher vibratory frequencies. The law of attraction and the manifestation process both depend on this idea.

Knowing how energy and vibrational frequency affect us and our health gives us the power to actively create and keep a balanced energy field. It motivates us to investigate techniques and equipment, such as essential oil use, that might help us maintain a healthy, energetic balance.

In the following parts, we shall explore using essential oils to affect and improve our energy states. By utilising their particular vibrational frequencies, we may intentionally work with essential oils to support energetic balance, healing, and general well-being.

Making Use of Essential Oils to Change Energy

Unique energetic qualities that essential oils have can affect our energy fields and support harmony and well-being. Each essential oil has a unique vibrational frequency from the plant from which it was harvested. It is thought that these qualities interact with our energetic systems to balance and improve energy flow inside our bodies and around us.

Citrus oils, including lemon, orange, and grapefruit, are renowned for their uplifting and energising properties. They can bolster vitality, release trapped energy, and uplift the spirit. Other energising oils that might increase mental clarity and attention include peppermint, rosemary, and eucalyptus.

Calming and Relaxing Oils: Some essential oils with calming and relaxing characteristics are lavender, chamomile, and ylang-ylang. These oils can foster a sense of calm and peace while reducing stress and anxiety. They frequently employ aromatherapy and relaxation techniques to foster emotional well-being and a calming environment.

Oils for Grounding and Balancing: Grounding and stabilising properties are well-known for essential oils, including patchouli, vetiver, and cedarwood. People who are disoriented or overwhelmed can use them to help them feel balanced and centred. These oils are frequently applied during meditation exercises to help people feel rooted and to anchor their energy.

Several essential oils, including frankincense, sage, and palo santo, have cleansing and purifying effects. They help remove bad energy, encourage emotional discharge, and establish sacred spaces. These oils are frequently used in rituals and ceremonies to enhance spiritual practises or purify the energy of a physical area.

How aromatherapy affects our energy systems

The vibrational frequencies of essential oils are thought to affect our energetic systems, such as our chakras, meridians, and aura. The following are a few ways that essential oils influence our active systems:

Chakras: The energy centers known as chakras are found along the central meridian of our body. Each chakra is linked to particular characteristics and oversees various bodily, emotional, and spiritual health facets. Specific essential oils can be chosen based on their related abilities to harmonise and align the chakras. For instance, applying rose oil to the heart chakra can encourage sentiments of compassion and love.

In traditional Chinese medicine, meridians are energy channels that run through the body, tying together numerous organs and systems. Physical and mental disorders may result from imbalances in these meridians. Specific acupressure spots along these meridians can be treated with essential oils to promote the passage of energy and reestablish balance.

Aura: It is thought that the electromagnetic field surrounding our body and containing information about our mental, emotional, and spiritual states is known as the aura. A harmonic and protective energy environment is created by purifying and bolstering the aura using essential oils. A robust and vivid aura can be achieved by diffusing essential oils or utilising them in energetic sprays.

Techniques for influencing energy with essential oils

Inhalation: Using essential oils to affect energy through inhalation is a popular and efficient technique. A diffuser can be filled with a few drops of essential oil, releasing the aroma into the air for inhalation. Alternatively, you can dab a drop of oil into your palms, cup your hands over your nose, and take deep breaths while doing so.

Topical application entails putting essential oils directly into the skin, which enables absorption and interaction with the body's energy systems. Before application, essential oils should be diluted with a carrier oil, like coconut or almond oil, to reduce the risk of skin reaction. The soles of the feet, wrists, and temples are a few examples of body parts that can be massaged because they are known to have energy points and meridian endpoints. Direct bloodstream absorption and energetic harmonisation are made possible by this method.

Bathing: A warm bath can relax and energise by adding a few drops of essential oil. The aroma surrounds you as you bathe in the oil-infused water, and the oils are absorbed through the skin. As you submerge yourself in the water, this approach encourages relaxation and gives the essential oils a chance to affect your energy field.

Spray bottles filled with purified water and essential oils make energetic sprays. Using this technique, you can spray the energy in your immediate surroundings and the area as a whole to create a calming, supportive, energetic environment. These sprays can eliminate stagnant energy from an area, cleanse and purify your aura, or improve your meditation and energy work.

Essential oils can be used to develop a connection with your energy and improve the experience during meditation and visualisation techniques. Before beginning your practice, you can either apply an oil to your pulse points that resonate with your intention or simply breathe deeply of the aroma. The aroma of the oil can strengthen your spiritual connection, anchor your focus, and quiet your mind.

Essential oils have been used in rituals and ceremonies for ages because of their strong energy qualities. They can be used to assist energetic shifts, create holy space, and call upon particular energies or deities. You can bring intention into the ceremony and boost the vibration of the venue by anointing yourself or objects with essential oils.

It is significant to remember that each person may have a different experience with essential oils and how they affect their energy. When choosing essential oils and experimenting with different methods, it is advised to follow your gut. Make adjustments to your practices based on how your body, emotions, and energy react to various oils.

To ensure their safety and effectiveness, it is vital to utilise pure, high-quality essential oils. Since essential oils are potent substances, some people may be sensitive to or allergic to particular oils. Before using any oil topically, perform a patch test, and if you have any concerns or unique medical issues, speak with a licenced aromatherapist or healthcare practitioner.

Essential oil usage can improve your general well-being, maintain energetic balance, and foster a closer relationship with both yourself and the environment around you. It can also be included in daily routines and energy practices. You may enable essential oils to have a beneficial effect on your energy and raise your vibratory frequency by actively utilising their energetic capabilities.

Making Energy Balance and Clear with Essential Oils

A fundamental idea in many spiritual and energetic practises the chakra system. According to popular belief, the body's core channel, which runs from the base of the spine to the top of the head, is comprised of spinning wheels or energy vortexes called chakras. Specific facets of our physical, emotional, and spiritual well-being are correlated with each chakra.

By balancing and harmonising the chakras, essential oils can encourage the best possible energy flow throughout the body. Here are some illustrations of essential oils that are frequently connected to each chakra:

Root Chakra (Muladhara): This chakra, which is situated at the base of the spine, is linked to security, stability, and a sense of grounding. Patchouli, vetiver, and cedarwood essential oils can support the root chakra's stability and balance.

Sacral Chakra (Svadhisthana): This chakra, which is located in the lower belly, is linked to creativity, sexuality, and emotional health. Jasmine, ylang-ylang, and orange essential oils can all help to balance the sacral chakra.

The Solar Plexus Chakra (Manipura), which is situated in the upper abdomen, is linked to one's own strength, self-assurance, and self-esteem. The solar plexus chakra can be balanced and stimulated with the use of essential oils like lemon, ginger, and bergamot.

Heart Chakra (Anahata): This chakra, which is located in the middle of the chest, is linked to emotions of love, compassion, and healing. Rose, lavender, and bergamot are a few examples of essential oils that can help the heart chakra become balanced.

Throat Chakra (Vishuddha): This chakra is situated in the area of the throat and is linked to self-expression, communication, and speaking one's truth. Essential oils like chamomile, peppermint, and eucalyptus can assist in balancing and energising the throat chakra.

Third Eye Chakra (Ajna): This chakra is related to intuition, perception, and spiritual consciousness. It is located in the middle of the forehead, just above the eyebrows. Frankincense, lavender, and clary sage are a few examples of essential oils that can help balance the third eye chakra.

Crown Chakra (Sahasrara): Situated at the top of the head, this chakra is linked to enlightenment, higher consciousness, and a connection to the spiritual world. Jasmine, lavender, and sandalwood essential oils, for example, can help to balance and open the crown chakra.

Apply the selected oil to the appropriate chakra area after diluting it in a carrier oil to employ essential oils for chakra balance. As an alternative, you can concentrate on the particular chakra and its corresponding qualities while diffusing the oil or inhaling it straight from the bottle.

Removing obstacles to the flow of positive energy

Stress, emotional difficulties, or environmental circumstances can cause negative energy to build up within our energetic field. It's critical to clear this energy if you want to be in a balanced, healthy state of being. Positive energy flow can be encouraged by using essential oils to purify and remove negative energy. The following are some applications for essential oils in this context:

Smudging: To make a smudging spray, mix distilled water with essential oils such as spanish sage, palo santo, and cedarwood, which are known for their purifying qualities. To eliminate negative energy from your body and your living area, spray the mixture around.

Warm baths can be infused with a few drops of essential oils like lavender, rosemary, or juniper. Imagine the water washing the bad energy from your body and aura while you soak. Allow yourself to unwind and release any pent-up or heavy energy while feeling refreshed and restored.

Space Clearing: To make a space-clearing spray, mix water or a neutral base like witch hazel with essential oils like lemon, tea tree, and peppermint. Focus on areas of your house or office that seem heavy or energetically stagnant while misting the mixture there.

Aura cleansing: Dilute essential oils like frankincense, rosemary, or lemongrass in a carrier oil before gently massaging your palms with the resulting mixture. Close your eyes and take a big breath in. Then, with your hands sweeping over your body from top to bottom, begin to visualise any negative energy being released and being replaced by positive, bright energy.

Setting up a calm setting will help with meditation and visualisation exercises. Use essential oils to create a relaxing environment by diffusing them, such as frankincense, sandalwood, or lavender. Imagine a bright white light encompassing your body while you meditate, clearing any unhealthy energy and recharging you with uplifting, healing energy.

Blends of essential oils for balancing and clearing the energy

You can combine the qualities of several oils to make essential oil blends that help general energetic balance and cleaning. Here are a few examples:

Lavender, sage, and lemon essential oils should be mixed in equivalence to create an energetic cleansing blend. This mixture encourages purification, frees energy that has become stuck and boosts the spirit. Use it as an energising spray or diffuse it in your space.

Grounding Blend: My personal favorite is the blend Balance**, a blend of Spruce, Ho Wood, Frankincense, Blue Tansy and Blue Chamomile. If you do not have that blend on hand, you can combine equal quantities of the essential oils of vetiver, patchouli, and cedarwood. This mixture encourages a sense of balance and grounding by helping to anchor and stabilise your energy. Apply it to the base of your spine or the soles of your feet after diluting it in carrier oil. Applying to your feet as a part of your daily routine will work wonders for your emotional balance, inadvertently raising your vibration.

Rose, bergamot, and clary sage essential oils should all be combined in an equal amounts to create the aura-balancing blend. This mixture supports emotional well-being and a positive energy flow by balancing and harmonising your aura. Apply it to your wrists or the area near your heart after diluting it in carrier oil. Other oils to balance and restore your aura are: spanish sage, lavender, Balance** and citrus oils from lemon or lime.

Create a blend using specific oils for each chakra, such as lavender for the crown chakra, ylang-ylang for the sacral chakra, and bergamot for the solar plexus chakra, to balance the chakras. Blend the oils together in a carrier oil in a ratio that feels instinctively balanced to you. During chakra balancing exercises, apply the blend to the respective chakra locations or diffuse it.

Trust your instinct when making essential oil blends, and modify the proportions of oils used to suit your preferences and needs. Always remember to appropriately dilute essential oils and run a patch test to check for any allergies or sensitivities.

When it comes to balancing and cleansing energy, essential oils can be strong allies. Essential oils provide a simple and accessible way to improve our energetic well-being, whether it's by assisting the chakra system, banishing bad energy, or using specialised blends for energetic cleansing. Our daily lives can be made more harmonic and balanced by implementing these techniques, which will help us feel more in tune with ourselves and the environment.

Aromatherapy for Mental and Emotional Energy

Our daily lives are significantly impacted by our emotions and mental health, which has an impact on our thoughts, behaviours, and general quality of life. Due to their strong and varied characteristics, essential oils have long been utilised to enhance mental and emotional health. In this section, we'll look at how essential oils can be used to control emotions, encourage emotional balance, improve concentration and mental clarity, and make mixes that are good for both the mind and the heart.

Using essential oils to promote emotional balance and manage emotions

Understanding emotions: Essential oils can be used as tools to manage and navigate emotions, which are a vital component of the human experience. Different oils have unique qualities that can assist emotional well-being and encourage the promotion of emotional balance, stress reduction, and relaxation.

A few essential oils with calming and grounding effects include vetiver, black spruce, lavender, chamomile, and bergamot. These oils can be used to manage stress and anxiety as well as to promote relaxation. To encourage emotional equilibrium, these oils can be directly applied, diffused, or inhaled.

Uplifting and energising oils: Oils with refreshing and energising qualities include citrus oils (such as lemon and orange) and uplifting flower oils (such as rose and jasmine). They can assist in boosting mood, encouraging optimism, and fending against low energy or depressive feelings.

The processing and discharge of emotions can be helped by using essential oils like frankincense, rosemary, and ylang-ylang. To aid in emotional healing and release, they can be added to baths, massages, and aromatherapy treatments.

Using essential oils to increase mental vigour, clarity, and focus

Enhancing focus, boosting cognitive function, and improving mental clarity are all possible benefits of using essential oils. The stimulating qualities of oils like Intune*, eucalyptus, peppermint, and rosemary help energise the mind and encourage mental alertness.

Memory and focus: Some essential oils, like those from lemon, basil, and sage, are believed to help memory retention and improve focus. To improve cognitive performance while doing work, studying, or other intellectually taxing activities, they can be diffused, breathed, or utilised in a personal inhaler.

Finding a balance between emotions and cognitive function can be made easier with the help of essential oils with grounding characteristics like vetiver and patchouli. They can aid in reducing mental tiredness, calming racing thoughts, and fostering steadiness and attention.

Mixtures of essential oils for mental and emotional health

Blend for reducing stress: Lavender, bergamot, and chamomile can be combined to provide a calming blend that can help with stress relief, relaxation, and emotional balance. Blend for focus and clarity: A combination of rosemary, peppermint, and lemon can assist in increasing mental clarity, memory recall, and alertness when performing jobs that call for concentration.

Combining uplifting floral oils like ylang-ylang and jasmine with citrus oils like orange and grapefruit can provide a revitalising blend that improves mood, encourages optimism, and enhances emotional well-being.

Grounding mixture: A grounding blend can be made by mixing essential oils such as vetiver, frankincense, and cedarwood. This blend encourages stability, clears the mind, and helps keep emotions in check.

Individuals respond to essential oils in different ways, and different people have varied tastes. It is advised to begin with tiny doses and increase or decrease according to sensitivity and response from the individual. Furthermore, for safe and efficient application, pure, high-quality essential oils must be used, together with the appropriate dilution techniques.

Essential Oils and Spiritual and Energetic Practises

Essential oils have a long history of being used in spiritual and energetic practises, providing a potent way to strengthen one's ties to the afterlife and raise one's vibrational frequency. This section will examine the use of essential oils for spiritual energy, enhancing energetic connections, boosting spiritual vibrations, and incorporating them into rituals, ceremonies, meditation, and mindfulness practices.

Using essential oils in mindfulness and meditation exercises

A path to inner calm, self-awareness, and spiritual development can be found through mindfulness and meditation practises. By encouraging relaxation, concentration, and a sense of sanctity, essential oils can significantly improve these practices. Essential oils can enhance the experience and promote a more profound connection to one's inner self and the present moment when used during meditation or mindfulness practises.

Essential oil inhalation: Using essential oils while meditating can be extremely beneficial. Essential oils' aromatic molecules have a direct effect on the limbic system, the brain's emotional centre, and can cause a range of emotional and spiritual reactions. Oils with grounding, relaxing, and centering qualities, such as frankincense, sandalwood, or lavender, are frequently used in aromatherapy.

Diffusion: Using a personal inhaler or diffusing essential oils in a room might help to set the mood for meditation. Essential oil mixes containing earthy, woodsy, or floral notes, such as cedarwood, patchouli, or rose, can promote calm and a sense of kinship with the divine.

Anointing: Before meditating, rubbing specific energy points or pulse points with essential oils will help you be more intentional and focused. For instance, applying a drop of a blend of essential oils to the heart center or third eye (between the brows) might improve intuition or open the heart to compassion and love.

Essential oil-based rituals and rites for spiritual energy

For centuries, people have used rituals and ceremonies to mark significant changes, establish spiritual connections, and pay respect to the sacred. By enhancing the energy and spiritual components of these practices, essential oils can increase their power and establish a sacred environment.

Cleaning and purification: White sage, palo santo, or cedarwood essential oils are frequently used in smudging ceremonies to drive away evil spirits and cleanse the area. It is thought that the fragrant smoke produced by these oils purifies and makes the environment suitable for spiritual work.

Consecration and anointing: Sacred items, ritual instruments, and even one's self can be anointed with essential oils to give them a sacred purpose and energy. Because of their sacred and purifying qualities, oils like frankincense, myrrh, rosemary, and jasmine are frequently utilised.

Sacred baths and foot soaks: A sacred and restorative experience can be created by incorporating a few drops of essential oils into a bath or foot soak. Lavender, rose, and frankincense oils, for example, can calm the mind, boost the spirit, and encourage a closer relationship with Source.

Using essential oils to strengthen energy ties and raise spiritual vibrations

Essential oils have the power to strengthen energy ties and boost spiritual vibrations, assisting people in their spiritual practices and creating a closer relationship with Source.

Balancing the chakras: Each chakra, or energy center, is linked to particular traits and spiritual dimensions. By balancing and aligning the chakras, essential oils can improve energy flow and promote spiritual development. For instance, applying ylang-ylang or rose oil to the heart chakra can encourage sentiments of compassion and love.

Healing through vibration: It's thought that each essential oil carries its own distinct vibrational frequency. Higher vibrational oils, like frankincense or rose, can be used to stimulate and raise one's own vibrational frequency, promoting spiritual development and connection.

Affirmations and intention setting: To increase the power of affirmations and intention setting, combine them with essential oils. People can increase the energetic resonance of their affirmations and aspirations by choosing essential oils that are in alignment with particular intents or traits they aim to foster, such as clarity, gratitude, or abundance.

Essential oils can also be utilised to establish energetic boundaries and provide protection. Because of its calming and shielding effects, oils like frankincense and black tourmaline are frequently used to help people keep their energy in check and protect themselves from draining influences.

Meditation and other spiritual exercises: Adding essential oils to your meditation or other spiritual exercises can enhance your experience and help you feel closer to God. Many sacred and spiritual oils, such as sandalwood, frankincense, and myrrh, aid people in reaching higher states of awareness and spiritual worlds.

It takes a lot of self-discovery and intuition to incorporate essential oils into spiritual and energy practises. It is crucial to make oil selections that align with one's goals, tastes, and unique energetic requirements. Exploration and experimentation are encouraged because every person may respond differently to various oils.

While essential oils can aid in spiritual and energetic practises, it is crucial to remember that they should not be used as a replacement for actual spiritual work, introspection, or the advice of a spiritual teacher or mentor. Although one's own intentions, commitment, and connection to the divine hold the ultimate transformational power, essential oils are instruments that can enrich and deepen the experience.

The use of essential oils in spiritual and energy practices has a long history. Essential oils can be effective allies in strengthening one's a spiritual path and connection to the divine, whether it is through rituals and ceremonies, improving energy connections and raising spiritual vibrations, or any combination of these. People can make holy spaces, amplify intentions, and promote their spiritual growth and change by actively using essential oils in these practices.

Utilising Essential Oils in Everyday Life

Enhancing well-being and encouraging a sense of balance and relaxation can be accomplished by including essential oils in personal care and self-care routines. Following are a few methods to use essential oils in your regular self-care routines:

Skincare: To address particular skin issues and encourage healthy-looking skin, you can incorporate essential oils into your skincare routine. Tea tree oil, for instance, has antimicrobial characteristics and can be applied as a spot treatment for skin that is prone to acne. For a calming effect, lavender oil can be used as a face oil or moisturiser. It is well renowned for its calming characteristics.

Taking a bath: You may make taking a warm bath a pleasurable and relaxing routine by adding a few drops of essential oil. For a soothing and stress-relieving bath, pick oils like lavender, chamomile, or ylang-ylang. An alternative is to take an energising bath with energising oils like peppermint or citrus oils.

Massage: Adding essential oils to massage therapy can increase the treatment's therapeutic and calming effects. Use a few drops of your favorite essential oil diluted in a carrier oil, like almond or jojoba oil, for a relaxing and fragrant massage. Eucalyptus or ginger essential oils may be helpful for reducing muscle tension and enhancing circulation.

Haircare: You can include essential oils in your haircare routine to hydrate the scalp, encourage strong hair growth, and give your locks more shine and scent. To stimulate the scalp and advance the health of your hair, think about using a few drops of rosemary oil in your shampoo. For a floral and upbeat scent, ylang-ylang oil can be used as a leave-in conditioner.

Using essential oils to create a positive atmosphere in the house

Our general well-being is greatly influenced by the environment we live in at home. We may encourage calmness, balance, and happiness by fostering an energy environment infused with essential oils. Here are some suggestions for using essential oils around the house:

Diffusing: A popular and efficient approach to spreading the aroma and therapeutic benefits of essential oils throughout your home is by using an essential oil diffuser. Select essential oils that are compatible with the ambience or energy you want to generate. Citrus oils like lemon or orange can boost and enliven the energy in a space, whereas lavender oil can encourage relaxation and a tranquil setting.

Room sprays: In a spray container, combine distilled water and essential oils to make your own natural room sprays. To freshen the space and add your preferred smell, spritz the mixture into the air. Oils of rosemary and peppermint can be combined to create an energising combination. Lavender and chamomile oils are effective for creating a tranquil environment.

Sprays for linens and fabrics: To lightly mist your linens, curtains, or cushions, add a few drops of essential oil to a spray bottle that is half-filled with water. This not only gives the materials a pleasing aroma but also infuses them with the oils' energising qualities. Use lavender or bergamot oil in the bedroom to create a calming atmosphere.

Candles for aromatherapy: For a double dosage of ambience and aromatherapy, choose candles produced from natural materials and blended with essential oils. When using candles, always use caution and never leave them unattended.

Using essential oils to increase overall vitality and wellbeing

Numerous essential oil practices can boost general energy and well-being in addition to self-care and fostering an energetic environment:

Morning energizer: To improve your mood and increase your energy levels, start your day with an energising essential oil blend. While getting ready for the day, diffuse energising oils such as citrus (lemon, lime, tangerine, orange, or grapefruit) or peppermint in your living environment. If you do not have a diffuser, you can create a

personal inhaler by adding a few drops of your preferred essential oil to a cotton wick.

Exercises for mindful breathing can be done with the help of essential oils to help you feel peaceful and relaxed. Pick oils with relaxing and grounding characteristics, like lavender, frankincense, or bergamot. Take slow, deep breaths while applying a drop of oil to your palms, rubbing them together, and cupping your hands over your nose. Allow the aroma to calm your body and mind as you concentrate on your breath.

Yoga and meditation: Incorporate essential oils into your routine to improve it. Before beginning your practice, apply a drop or two of your favourite oil on the back of your neck or your wrists. As an alternative, you can make your own yoga mat spray by mixing water, witch hazel, and aromatic oils. Before each yoga class, spray your mat to create a calm and uplifting environment.

Create a relaxing nighttime routine to encourage relaxation and good sleep. To create a peaceful atmosphere, diffuse calming essential oils in your bedroom, such as lavender, chamomile, or sandalwood. These oils can also be used to make a linen spray to mist your bedding before bed or to add a drop to your pillow. Allow the soothing perfume to settle your mind for a time so that you can get ready for a peaceful night's sleep.

Clearing your energy: Use essential oils to purify and clear your area and your own energy. Smudging and cleansing negative energy frequently involve the use of sage, palo santo, or cedarwood essential oils. Use your selected oil as a room spray or mist to clean and revitalise your surroundings by diluting a few drops of it with water. A crystal or gemstone essence that resonates with you can be combined with water, essential oils, and other ingredients to make a personal aura spray.

When choosing and utilising essential oils, it is advised to pay attention to your body and intuition because individual reactions to the oils can differ. If you have any questions or certain health conditions, it's important to do your research and speak with a trained aromatherapist or healthcare expert. Some oils may have contraindications or sensitivities for some people.

Using essential oils regularly can be a pleasurable and successful approach to increasing general vitality and well-being. You have the chance to harness the power of these organic essences to improve your vitality, balance your energy, and develop a deeper feeling of self-care and connection, whether through personal care routines, designing an energetic environment, or particular essential oil practices.

We have discovered a variety of possible advantages that these organic materials may provide during our investigation into using essential oils to harness energy. Essential oils have the power to significantly impact our energetic well-being by changing our vibrational frequency and fostering harmony and balance both within us and around us.

Emotional equilibrium can be promoted by using essential oils for energy, which is one of their main advantages. Some essential oils, including chamomile and lavender, have relaxing effects that can calm the mind and reduce tension. Other oils, such as peppermint and citrus oils, are well known for their uplifting properties, which help elevate mood and increase cheerfulness.

Additionally, essential oils may improve concentration and mental clarity. Lemon and rosemary oils, for example, help energise the mind and enhance cognitive function, enhancing focus and productivity. These essential oils help improve mental energy and encourage clear, concentrated thinking in our daily lives.

Additionally, essential oils can benefit our spiritual health. Long utilised in spiritual practices, oils like frankincense and sandalwood are renowned for their capacity to heighten spiritual vibrations, deepen meditation, and foster a sense of connectedness. We may foster a climate that encourages our spiritual development and discovery by including these oils in our spiritual rituals and practises.

Additionally, using essential oils can help us to balance and purify our energies. We can encourage the harmonious flow of energy throughout our bodies by using essential oils that resonate with particular chakras or energy centres. Additionally, essential oils can be utilised for energetic cleansing, which aids in removing any bad or sluggish energy and encouraging the flow of good energy.

Encouragement to research and test using essential oils for energy harvesting

As we come to a conclusion in our investigation of essential oils and their function in generating energy, it is critical to inspire people to set out on their own discovery and experimenting trips. Each person's experience with essential oils is different, and the only way to find the oils that most profoundly align with their energetic requirements and aspirations is via personal investigation.

The usage of essential oils is advised to be approached with an open mind and a readiness to trust one's instincts. Understanding how essential oils impact our energy and general well-being can be gained by experimenting with various oils, blends, and application techniques. We can develop a stronger connection with ourselves, our environment, and the energetic qualities of essential oils by embracing this journey of self-discovery.

It is crucial to keep in mind that using essential oils to boost energy should be considered an additional practice rather than a replacement for expert medical or psychological treatment. Before introducing essential oils into your routine, it is always advised to speak with a healthcare professional or licenced aromatherapist if you have any underlying health disorders or concerns.

An effective and convenient instrument for generating energy and enhancing our energetic well-being is provided by essential oils. Essential oils have the power to raise our vibratory frequency and overall energy, whether it is through the fragrant advantages of inhalation, the healing effects of topical application, or the spiritual and emotional support they offer.

We are able to build a greater feeling of balance, harmony, and vigour in our life thanks to the energetic characteristics of essential oils in conjunction with our intention and attention. By using essential oils, we can strengthen our energetic connection, boost emotional well-being, and foster spiritual development by drawing upon the knowledge of nature and the potency of aroma.

The decision to use essential oils for energy is ultimately a personal one. Each person has the freedom to investigate, test, and discover their own method of using these organic materials. So embrace the transforming potential of essential oils, believe in your gut, and give them time.

Chapter 2: What is vibrational frequency?

The rate at which an object or a system oscillates or vibrates is referred to as its vibrational frequency. The frequency of a wave or vibrating particle is described using this fundamental idea from physics. Vibrational frequency, to put it simply, gauges how swiftly or slowly something vibrates or oscillates.

Everything in the universe, including our bodies, is constituted of energy when viewed from the perspective of humans. This energy vibrates at a variety of frequencies and is never motionless. Each material or item has a distinct vibrational frequency that can be expressed in hertz (Hz). The pace at which an object's atoms and molecules move or vibrate determines its vibrational frequency.

The Vibrations and Energy Theory

It is essential to appreciate the idea of energy in order to comprehend vibrational frequency. All physical, chemical, and biological processes are propelled by energy. It can be found in a variety of forms, including kinetic energy (the energy of motion), potential energy, thermal energy, electromagnetic energy, and energy stored in the form of heat.

The way energy appears at the atomic and molecular levels is through vibrations. Atoms and molecules are constantly in motion rather than being static objects. They move, rotate, and vibrate, generating waves of energy. Electromagnetic fields, the building blocks of energy and vibration, are produced by these waves.

Vibrational Frequency and General Well-Being: A Relationship

Beyond the boundaries of physics, the idea of vibrational frequency affects our general well-being. Every living thing has an energetic frequency, according to proponents of alternative healing treatments and spiritual beliefs, and maintaining a balanced and harmonic frequency is crucial for optimum health and well-being.

According to this viewpoint, we feel a feeling of balance, vitality, and emotional well-being when our vibrational frequency is in tune. On the other side, if our vibrational frequency is interrupted or out of harmony, it can cause a variety of mental, emotional, and physical illnesses.

Based on the premise that various vibrational frequencies have various effects on the body and psyche of people, there is a correlation between vibrational frequency and general well-being. Higher frequencies are regarded to be linked to good feelings, mental acuity, and spiritual connection, whereas lower frequencies are thought to be linked to stress, illness, and negativity.

Examples of high-frequency emotions that resonate at a higher vibratory frequency include love, joy, and appreciation. These feelings are thought to support general health, immunological function, and well-being. Contrarily, low-frequency emotions like fear, wrath, and tension are thought to disturb the body's normal energy flow and cause a number of health problems if they persist.

Vibrational frequency proponents contend that outside forces have an impact on our energetic equilibrium. Our vibratory frequency may be lowered by environmental factors like exposure to poisons, electromagnetic radiation, and unfavourable emotions from others. On the other hand, practising positivity-enhancing activities like meditation, spending time in nature, and listening to upbeat music can raise our vibrational frequency and improve our general well-being.

Research in the area of psychoneuroimmunology has recently looked into how stress, emotions, and physical health are related. There is a rising acknowledgement of the mind-body connection and the impact of emotions on health outcomes, even if scientific understanding of the vibrational frequency and its direct impact on wellbeing is still in its early stages.

The rate at which an object or system oscillates or vibrates is referred to as its vibrational frequency. It affects our general well-being and is a key idea in physics. We can better understand the importance of vibrational frequency in our daily lives if we have a basic understanding of energy and vibrations. There is a growing understanding of the role of emotions and energy in health outcomes, even if more research is required to completely understand the mechanisms underlying the association between vibrational frequency and general well-being. Investigating techniques that encourage a harmonious and balanced vibrational frequency may open up fresh possibilities for improving well-being and advancing holistic health.

The Vibrational Frequency of Essential Oils

Essential oils are potent, aromatic molecules that are extracted from the flowers, leaves, stems, bark, and roots of plants. They are obtained using procedures like solvent extraction, cold-press extraction, and steam distillation. These oils capture the distinct essence and advantageous traits of plants, such as their aroma and therapeutic effects. Due to their intense and varied effects, essential oils have been utilised for ages in traditional medicine, perfumery, and even spiritual practices.

The Process Used to Make Essential Oils from Plants

Understanding that everything in the cosmos, including plants and people, is made up of energy vibrating at different frequencies is crucial to comprehending the vibrational frequency of essential oils. Because they are made from plants, essential oils have their own vibrational frequencies. It is thought that those who engage with these oils will experience changes in their bodily, emotional, and spiritual health as a result of this vibrational energy.

Factors Affecting the Essential Oils' Vibrational Frequency

Plant Species: The vibrational frequencies of various plant species vary, which affects how strongly their essential oils resonate. For instance, the vibrational frequency of lavender essential oil differs from that of eucalyptus essential oil.

Environmental Factors: The vibrational frequency of the plant and, consequently, the essential oil it produces can be influenced by the environment in which it grows, including elements like soil quality, climate, and altitude.

Methods of Harvesting and Processing: The vibrational frequency of the essential oil can be affected by the methods used to collect and process the plants. The vibrational integrity of the oil is best preserved using gentle and non-destructive techniques.

Individual Characteristics: Some people think that an essential oil's vibrational frequency can also be affected by the personality traits and level of consciousness of the person who is extracting or using it.

The Vibrational Frequency of Essential Oils: Research and Studies

Essential oil vibrational frequency research is still in its infancy, and much of what is known about it comes from vibrational medicine, energy healing, and anecdotal data. Even though there haven't been many studies explicitly looking at the vibrational frequency of essential oils, interest is developing in this field. Related aspects have been investigated in some studies and observations:

Bioelectrography: Gas discharge visualisation, commonly referred to as bioelectrography, has been utilised to examine the energy emissions from essential oils. Through this method, the energy field surrounding the oils is captured, and its vibrational frequency patterns are revealed.

Kirlian photography has been used to examine and record the ethereal energy fields that essential oils emit. The vibrational frequencies connected to various oils can be represented visually using these graphics.

Assessments using intuition and energy: Many practitioners and others with training in energy healing methods examine the vibrational frequency of essential oils using their intuition and energy. Despite their subjectivity, these evaluations can provide insightful information about the oils' energetic properties.

The effects of essential oils on emotional health and energy levels have been the subject of numerous research. These studies offer circumstantial proof of the oils' capacity to affect people's energy states despite not explicitly measuring vibrational frequency.

The vibrational frequency of essential oils continues to be a subject of interest within the holistic and alternative medicine communities, despite the fact that research in this area is still being conducted. Our knowledge of the energetic properties of essential oils is constantly growing as a result of research into vibrational medicine and future uses.

Essential oils have unique vibrational frequencies that can affect the health of people who engage with them. Numerous variables, including plant species, ambient circumstances, harvesting and processing techniques, and individual attributes, have an impact on the vibrational frequency of essential oils. There is developing research and observations that offer insights into this field, despite the fact that there hasn't been much scientific study precisely on the vibrational frequency of essential oils.

Bioelectrography, sometimes referred to as gas discharge visualisation, is one method for examining the vibrational frequency of essential oils. Using this method, the energy emissions from essential oils are captured, and the energy field around the oils is examined. The patterns and traits of the energy releases can provide researchers with information on the vibrational frequency of the oils.

Another method for observing and capturing the ethereal energy fields that essential oils create is Kirlian photography. This kind of photography records the corona or energy discharge that surrounds an object. The energetic properties of essential oils can be visualised using Kirlian photos, which may also reveal information about their vibrational frequency.

Many practitioners and people educated in energy healing techniques also rely on intuitive and energetic assessments to determine the vibrational frequency of essential oils in addition to these scientific methodologies. In these evaluations, the energetic properties of the oils are perceived and analysed, utilising one's intuition and sensitivity to subtle energy. Even though they are inherently subjective, these evaluations can offer important details on the energy effects and vibrational frequency of essential oils.

Numerous research has also examined the energy and emotional impacts of essential oils. These studies offer circumstantial proof of the oils' capacity to affect people's energy states despite not explicitly measuring vibrational frequency. For instance, it has been discovered that some essential oils encourage relaxation, lessen stress, and improve mood. The vibrational frequency of the oils and their capacity to interact with the human energy field are thought to be responsible for these emotional and energetic impacts.

Even though there hasn't been much scientific study on the vibrational frequency of essential oils, the growing popularity of vibrational medicine and energy healing points to a possible connection between essential oils and their vibrational properties. The idea that essential oils have distinctive vibrational frequencies that can affect the subtle energies of the body and mind is supported by the fact that many people and practitioners report experiencing energetic changes and beneficial effects while working with essential oils.

It is crucial to remember that essential oils' vibrational frequencies should not be considered in isolation when analysing their medicinal effects. A rich blend of chemical components found in essential oils contributes to their overall qualities and advantages. You could think of vibrational frequency as another dimension that communicates with the person's energetic system.

Essential oils contain unique vibrational frequencies that might affect a person's health. There is developing research and observations that offer insights into this field, despite the fact that there hasn't been much scientific study precisely on the vibrational frequency of essential oils.

Intuitive and energetic assessments, Kirlian photography, bio electrography, and other methods are used to investigate and assess the vibrational frequency of essential oils. Indirect evidence for this interaction between essential oils and the subtle energies of the body and mind can also be found in studies on the emotional and energetic impacts of essential oils. Our knowledge of the energetic properties of essential oils and their potential uses in promoting holistic well-being can be furthered by additional research in this area.

Essential Oils' Effects on Vibrational Frequency

Effects of essential oils on the vibrational frequency of people:

The relationship between smell and feelings:

Our sense of smell is intimately connected to our feelings and can significantly affect our mood, well-being, and overall vibrational frequency. Certain smells can elicit particular feelings and cause people to react positively or negatively. The use of essential oils to affect vibrational frequency is based on the relationship between aroma and emotions.

The limbic system in the brain is intimately tied to the olfactory system, which is stimulated when we inhale the aroma of essential oils. Processing of emotions, memories, and hormone reactions occurs in the limbic system. Because of this, essential oils have the power to cause emotional and physical changes that alter our vibrational frequency.

The potential advantages of utilising essential oils for vibrational frequency balance include the following:

Numerous advantages can be had by using essential oils in terms of harmonising and raising vibrational frequency. Potential benefits include the following:

a. Stress reduction: relaxing essential oils like bergamot, chamomile, and lavender offer a relaxing effect that can aid with anxiety and stress reduction. These oils can aid in restoring a healthy vibrational frequency by encouraging a sense of calm.

b. Enhancement of mood: Certain essential oils, such as peppermint and citrus oils (such as lemon, orange, and grapefruit), offer uplifting and energising properties. They can elevate vibrational frequency, elevate positivity, and elevate mood.

c. Emotional healing: Rose, ylang-ylang, and frankincense are a few essential oils that have traditionally been used for this purpose. They can encourage self-love, enhance emotional well-being, and aid in the removal of emotional blockages, which eventually alter vibrational frequency. Certain essential oils and the vibrational frequencies they are connected with:

Examples of essential oils with high vibrational frequencies

Essential oils with high vibrational frequencies are thought to resonate with higher energy states, fostering spiritual and emotional development. Several instances include:

Frankincense: With a high vibrational frequency, frankincense is renowned for its contemplative and spiritual benefits. It is frequently employed in spiritual practises to strengthen ties and foster a sense of inner tranquilly.

Rose: Rose essential oil is linked to higher consciousness, love, and compassion. Its high vibrational frequency can promote sentiments of love, harmony, and forgiveness by opening the heart chakra.

Lavender: The relaxing and balancing properties of lavender essential oil are well known. It has a calming vibrational frequency that encourages calmness, relaxation, and a feeling of well-being.

Examples of essential oils with low vibrational frequencies

Essential oils with a low vibrational frequency are supposed to have a grounding effect and can be used to deal with troubling emotions or encourage stability. Several instances include:

Patchouli: The earthy, grounding aroma of patchouli essential oil is well-known. It is thought to provide a sense of stability and security while assisting in the release of negative emotions and anxiety.

Vetiver: Used for centring and grounding, vetiver essential oil has a rich, smokey aroma. It can help to promote mental stability, relieve stress, and calm an overworked mind.

Myrrh: The anchoring and defence properties of myrrh essential oil are accompanied by its rich, pleasant aroma. It helps facilitate emotional recovery and foster a sense of stability in spiritual practises.

We may harness their potential advantages and raise our overall vibrational frequency by using these high or low-vibrational frequency essential oils in our daily routines. It's crucial to keep in mind that everyone's experiences with essential oils will be unique, so it's best to pick scents that appeal to you personally and match your own energy.

It's important to keep in mind that an essential oil's vibrational frequency is not exclusively influenced by its perfume or scent when utilising them to balance vibrational frequency. The vibrational frequency of the oil can also be affected by elements, including the oil's composition, the process used to extract it, and the overall intention and energy used when using it.

It is advised to practise mindfulness and intention-based activities to increase the benefits of essential oils on vibrational frequency. The vibrational impact of using essential oils can be enhanced by establishing clear intentions, cultivating gratitude, including meditation or energy healing practises, and practising these practises concurrently.

To guarantee the maximum vibrational frequency, it is also crucial to choose pure, high-quality essential oils. Oils that have been diluted or made from synthetic fragrances could not have the same energising properties as pure essential oils. Seek out trustworthy vendors who are upfront about the oils' sourcing, extraction processes, and quality.

It's important to keep in mind that when it comes to essential oils, individual tastes and sensitivities can vary. One person's solution could not have the same impact on another. It is crucial to investigate and test out various oils in order to identify ones that resonate with your personal vibrational frequency.

There are several ways to incorporate essential oils into your everyday routine:

One of the most popular ways to use essential oils is by inhalation. An aromatherapy diffuser can be used to spread the scent of the oils throughout the space. As an alternative, you can inhale directly from the bottle or apply a few drops of essential oil to a tissue. Breathe deeply, allowing the aroma to fill your senses and raise your vibrational frequency.

Topical application: Essential oils may be applied topically to particular body parts after being diluted with a carrier oil, such as almond or coconut oil. Vibrational frequency can be balanced by applying oils to energy centres or acupressure sites, such as the wrists, temples, or heart chakra. To be sure that your skin will tolerate the oil, it's advised to follow the correct dilution instructions and conduct a patch test.

When taking a bath, a few drops of essential oil can make the water calming and fragrant. The essential oils can permeate your skin and arouse your senses while you submerge yourself in the water, aiding in relaxation and balancing your vibrational frequency.

Energy healing techniques and meditation: Using essential oils in conjunction with energy healing techniques or meditation can boost their effectiveness. You can intensify your experience and boost your vibrational frequency by applying oils to specific body parts, utilising them during

Reiki or other energy healing treatments, or anointing yourself with oils before or after meditation.

When employing essential oils to affect the vibrational frequency, as with any holistic method, it's crucial to keep an open mind and pay attention to your body's reaction. Pay note of how each oil makes you feel, how much energy you have, and how you feel overall. Honour your intuition and stop using oil if it doesn't seem right to you or has a negative effect.

Essential oils' ability to affect emotions, encourage balance, and boost general well-being can have a substantial impact on vibrational frequency. Essential oils can influence our vibrational frequency due to the association between smell and emotions, which makes them effective instruments for spiritual and personal development.

We can take advantage of the special abilities of particular essential oils with high or low vibrational frequencies, such as frankincense, rose, lavender, patchouli, vetiver, or myrrh, by selecting them. It is crucial to utilise essential oils with intention, attention, and a focus on self-exploration, as each person will have different experiences and preferences.

How to Change Vibrational Frequency with Essential Oils

Since ancient times, people have employed essential oils for their therapeutic benefits and capacity to improve well-being. The vibrational frequency of essential oils, which relates to a substance's energetic resonance, is one of their most intriguing characteristics. People can use essential oils to build harmony and balance within themselves by learning how to use them to affect the vibrational frequency and putting those skills to use.

Inhalation, topical application, and additional techniques like utilising them in baths or incorporating them into energy healing or meditation practises the three major ways that essential oils are used for this purpose and are covered in this article.

Inhalation

One of the most popular and efficient methods for using essential oils to affect vibrational frequency is inhalation. The scent molecules of essential oils interact with the olfactory system when they are breathed, causing a variety of physiological and emotional reactions.

Aromatizing with essential oils

Using an essential oil diffuser to spread the oil particles into the air is how essential oils are diffused. By using this technique, the perfume can fill the entire space and produce a relaxing and healing atmosphere. Diffusing essential oils helps respiratory health and emotional well-being in addition to raising the vibrational frequency of the environment. Selecting essential oils that correspond with your desired results is crucial because different essential oils have different effects.

Adopting direct inhalation methods

Direct inhalation entails taking a breath of essential oils straight from the bottle or a portable inhaler. This technique enables a swift and focused effect while offering a more concentrated sensation of the oil's aroma. Simply place the bottle or inhaler next to your nose to use direct inhalation. Then, inhale deeply. This method is especially beneficial for fostering present-moment calm, relaxation, or emotional equilibrium.

Application to the Skin

Topical application is applying essential oils directly to the skin, allowing for absorption and interaction with acupressure points and the body's energy centres. Important to keep in mind is that essential oils should be thoroughly diluted before applying to the skin because they are highly concentrated.

Guidelines for safe usage and dilution:

Before administering essential oils topically, they are often diluted with carrier oil, such as coconut oil or jojoba oil. This ensures that the oil is distributed uniformly throughout the skin surface and lowers the chance of skin irritation. According to general dilution rules, adults should mix 1-3 drops of essential oil per teaspoon of carrier oil, while kids and people with sensitive skin should use a lower dilution ratio.

Applying essential oils to particular acupressure or energy points:

Chakras, or energy centers, are thought to be concentrated concentrations of energy in the body. Specific locations throughout the body's energy meridians are called acupressure sites. The vibrational frequency of essential oils can have a direct impact on the body's energy flow and equilibrium by applying them to certain locations. Putting peppermint oil in the solar plexus chakra (placed in the upper abdomen) can help boost vitality and confidence, while putting lavender oil in the crown chakra (located at the top of the head) may encourage a sense of serenity and spiritual connection.

Other Techniques

There are additional ways to use essential oils to affect vibrational frequency than inhalation and topically. These approaches offer extra chances to include essential oils in daily activities and self-care routines.

Using essential oils during bathing:

A warm bath can be made more relaxing and pleasant by adding a few drops of essential oils, which diffuse in the water. Warm water and essential oils work together to promote relaxation, reduce stress, and raise the body's and mind's overall vibratory frequency.

Using essential oils for energy work or meditation:

Essential oils can be effective allies in energy healing and meditation techniques. Essential oils can heighten the vibrational frequency and enrich the experience when used in conjunction with these techniques.

Essential oils can be applied directly to pulse points before beginning a meditation session or diffused throughout the room. An environment that is peaceful and concentrated, thanks to the oils' scent, can facilitate a deeper level of meditation. Selecting oils that encourage calm, clarity or spiritual connection can enhance the advantages of meditating because different oils may have diverse effects on the mind and emotions.

Similar to this, essential oils can be applied to the body or diffused in the treatment room in energy healing techniques like Reiki or acupuncture. The body's energy flow can be balanced and harmonised with the aid of oils, improving the efficacy of the therapeutic session. To support the desired therapeutic effects, practitioners may use essential oils that are correlated with particular energy centers or meridian pathways.

It's crucial to keep in mind that each person's reaction to essential oils may be different. Therefore it's advised to explore and follow your body's intuition while utilising them for meditation or energy healing techniques. Additionally, getting personalised advice based on particular needs and objectives can be obtained by speaking with a qualified essential emotions coach, certified essential oil practitioner or aromatherapist.

There are numerous chances to favourably affect vibrational frequency by including essential oils in everyday routines, and self-care practises. Essential oils offer a natural and holistic approach to boosting overall well-being, whether through inhalation, topical use, or other techniques like bathing or meditation.

It's critical to take into account the following advice to maximise the advantages and safety of utilising essential oils:

Invest in high-quality essential oils: Look for oils that are unadulterated, organic, and devoid of artificial ingredients. Look for trustworthy companies that are open about their sourcing and testing procedures.

Before using essential oils topically, conduct a patch test on a small area of the skin to check for any potential sensitivities or allergies. Then, thoroughly dilute the essential oils. To prevent skin sensitivity, dilute essential oils with carrier oil as needed.

Observe usage instructions: Each essential oil has specific recommendations for use. Some oils could be more strong than others, requiring less dilution or less time for inhalation. Learn the particular recommendations for each oil and make the necessary adjustments.

Pay attention to how your body and mind react to various oils and application techniques. Everyone will likely have a different experience with essential oils, so trust your gut and tailor your strategy to your particular requirements and preferences.

Utilising essential oils to alter vibrational frequency is a holistic and all-natural way to encourage harmony and well-being. A harmonious vibrational frequency can be achieved through inhalation via diffusion or direct inhalation, topical application with appropriate dilution and targeting of particular energy centers, and the use of essential oils in rituals like bathing, meditation, or energy healing. People can make use of the potential of essential oils to improve their general well-being and lead more balanced and meaningful lives by learning about and experimenting with these techniques.

We have looked at the idea of vibrational frequency and how it relates to our health throughout this discussion. Everything in the cosmos vibrates at a certain rate, including our thoughts, feelings, and physical bodies, which is referred to as vibrational frequency. It is thought that sustaining a harmonious and balanced vibrational frequency might support overall well-being.

When we encounter unpleasant emotions or thoughts, our vibrational frequency may become unbalanced or lower since our ideas and emotions emanate particular frequencies. Positive feelings and thoughts, on the other hand, might increase our vibrational frequency. Plant-derived essential oils are known to have their own distinct vibrational frequencies. We may change our vibrational frequency to support balance and well-being by using essential oils.

Understanding and using essential oils for vibrational frequency is important:

It's crucial to comprehend and use essential oils for vibrational frequency for a number of reasons. First off, essential oils have been used for their medicinal benefits across a variety of civilizations for ages. We may harness their potential to have a favourable effect on our emotional, mental, and physical states by incorporating them into our daily lives.

The vibrational frequencies of essential oils can interact with and affect our own vibrational frequencies. We may increase our own vibrational frequency and encourage a happier frame of mind by using oils with higher vibrational frequencies. This may result in an uplifted mood, more energy, and an improvement in general well-being.

Additionally, essential oils can be utilised as self-care and self-healing techniques. In addition to helping us to treat imbalances and promote our body's natural healing processes, they offer a natural and comprehensive approach to wellness. Incorporating essential oils into our daily routines can assist us in maintaining a more balanced and raised vibrational frequency, whether by inhalation, topical application, or other techniques.

Encouragement for additional investigation and testing:

It is crucial to promote additional investigation and experimentation in this area as we draw to a close to our investigation of vibrational frequency and essential oils. There is still much to study and learn about when it comes to the vibrational frequency of essential oils and their potential impacts on human well-being.

It is crucial for each person to identify the essential oils that speak to them personally because everyone's experiences with essential oils might differ. People can find precise oils that raise their vibrational frequency and meet their own needs by experimenting and exploring.

It is important to keep conducting scientific studies to learn more about how essential oils affect vibrational frequency. This can provide us with a fuller knowledge of the processes that underlie how essential oils interact with our vibrational frequencies and how they might be used therapeutically.

Understanding and using essential oils can be a potent tool in promoting balance and harmony since vibrational frequency has a key influence on our general well-being. We may improve our emotional, mental, and physical states and change the vibrational frequency of our bodies by introducing essential oils into our daily life. Let's embrace the potential of essential oils, learn more about their advantages, and set off on a quest for introspection and holistic wellness.

Chapter 3: What are the benefits of raising your vibrational frequency?

Living a full and balanced life requires improving emotional well-being. Numerous advantages that improve our emotional condition occur when we increase our vibrational frequency. The three major benefits of increasing one's vibrational frequency—increased happiness and optimism, less stress and anxiety, and enhanced emotional resilience and problem-solving skills—are examined in this article.

Increased Joy and Positivity:

Increasing our vibrational frequency encourages a change in our perspective and emotional state, which increases happiness and positivity. We become more in tune with joy, gratitude, and love when we work at a higher frequency. This change enables us to live life with a more positive view and to appreciate the gifts and beauty all around us. We gain a deeper sense of contentment as we become more conscious of the current moment.

We can elevate our emotions and decide to concentrate on the good things in life by actively elevating our vibrational frequency. This positive energy draws more positive things and people into our life, starting a positive feedback loop that makes us feel good.

Stress and anxiety levels are reduced:

Increasing our vibrational frequency can also help us feel less stressed and anxious. We are more vulnerable to stressful situations and bad emotions when we are operating at a lower frequency. However, we can more effectively control stress and anxiety by actively raising our frequency.

A greater sense of inner peace and tranquillity is related to higher vibrational levels. Our ability to overcome obstacles increases when we get a wider perspective and find it simpler to step back from trying circumstances. Raising our vibratory frequency helps us let go of unhelpful thought patterns, anxieties, and fears, which makes us feel lighter and freer.

Increased Emotional Resilience and Challenge Handling Capability:

Raising our vibratory frequency strengthens our emotional fortitude and gives us the tools we need to deal with difficulties more skillfully. We develop a positive mindset that enables us to face challenges with better clarity and composure when we work at a higher frequency.

We strengthen our ties to our inner wisdom and intuition by increasing our vibrational frequency. As a result of our increased awareness, we are better able to deal with difficult circumstances and make decisions that are in line with our true selves. When faced with difficulty, we are able to retain emotional balance and become less reactive to outside factors.

Additionally, elevating our vibrational frequency improves our ability to take care of and be compassionate towards ourselves. We become more aware of our own needs, establishing sound boundaries and placing our well-being first. With this self-nurturing strategy, we can overcome obstacles and setbacks with greater fortitude and perseverance.

There are several advantages to improving our vibrational frequency in order to improve our emotional well-being, including an increase in positivity and happiness, a decrease in stress and anxiety, and an increase in emotional resilience. We can feel more joy and contentment if we intentionally change our perspective and concentrate on the good things in life. Additionally, when our vibration increases, we gain the capacity to handle stress more skillfully and approach problems with more clarity and serenity. This journey to better emotional health gives us the power to lead more fruitful, balanced lives.

Physical Fitness and Energy

A meaningful and successful life depends on maintaining good physical health. The importance of overall well-being, which includes increasing one's vibrational frequency, is becoming increasingly understood, in contrast to traditional healthcare techniques that prioritise treating diseases and symptoms. This post will discuss how increasing your vibrational frequency can enhance your physical well-being. We'll talk specifically about a strengthened immune system, better general health, more vigor and energy, and quicker recovery from diseases and injuries.

Enhanced Immunity and Better Health Overall:

The improvement of your immune system is a big advantage of increasing your vibrational frequency. The body's defence mechanism against hazardous germs, bacteria, and viruses is the immune system. Your immune system responds to possible threats more effectively and robustly when your vibrational frequency is raised.

Reducing the effects of stress is one way that increasing your vibrational frequency strengthens your immune system. Chronic stress impairs immunity, increasing your susceptibility to disease. However, you may lessen the harmful impacts of stress and advance general health by increasing your vibrational frequency. An immune system that is more balanced and resilient is a result of increased optimism, emotional fortitude, and decreased worry.

Additionally, increasing your vibrational frequency encourages leading a healthy lifestyle. When you are operating at a higher frequency, you are drawn to pursuits that enhance your well-being, such as consistent exercise, wholesome food, and adequate rest. Your immune system will benefit from these behaviours, which will also boost your general health.

Increased Vitality and Energy Levels:

Your energy and vitality can be significantly affected by increasing your vibrational frequency. The chakras and meridians, as well as the body's energetic system as a whole, are all tightly related to vibrational frequency. Your energy flow becomes stagnate when your vibrational frequency is low, which causes you to feel worn out, lethargic, and devoid of vigour. But when your vibrational frequency rises, your body's energy starts to move more freely and harmoniously.

You can access a source of energy that makes you feel more energetic and alive by increasing your vibrational frequency. Increased productivity, sharper attention, and a better capacity for physical activity are all results of this enhanced energy. Given that you have more energy and the capacity and passion to engage in physical activities, you might discover that you are naturally driven to hobbies, physical activities, and endeavours.

Faster Recovery from Illnesses and Accidents:

Raising your vibrational frequency has the ability to speed up the healing and recovery process, which is a tremendous advantage. The body's equilibrium is frequently upset by illnesses and injuries, leading to physical imbalances and suffering. However, by increasing your vibrational frequency, you help your body achieve a state of balance and harmony, which aids and hastens the healing process.

Cellular regeneration and repair are encouraged by increasing vibrational frequency. Specific frequencies are used by the body's cells to vibrate. Therefore when your overall vibrational frequency is raised, it has a favourable impact on the vibration of individual cells. This phenomenon can help the body's own regenerative processes function more effectively while also repairing damaged tissues and lowering inflammation.

Additionally, increasing your vibrational frequency can benefit your mental and emotional health, which in turn determines how quickly your body heals physically. You may foster a healing atmosphere by lowering stress, anxiety, and unpleasant feelings. Studies have revealed that people with optimistic attitudes and mental states typically heal from procedures, wounds, and illnesses more quickly.

There are several advantages to increasing your vibrational frequency for your physical health and vigour. You can experience a stronger immune system, greater general health, more vitality, and quicker healing and recovery from diseases or injuries by achieving a condition of balance and harmony within your body. All of these advantages work together to promote comprehensive well-being.

You become better able to fend off infections and preserve good health when your immune system is bolstered by increasing your vibrational frequency. Fighting off pathogens, germs, and viruses that can cause illnesses and diseases requires a strong immune system. Raising your vibrational frequency boosts the immune system's capacity to work effectively and efficiently by lowering stress levels and encouraging emotional resilience.

Raising your vibrational frequency also improves your general health in addition to strengthening your immune system. When you are operating at a higher frequency, you are drawn to making good lifestyle decisions like regular exercise, a balanced diet, and enough sleep. These behaviours help people keep a healthy weight, which lowers their chance of developing chronic illnesses, including diabetes, cardiovascular problems, and some types of cancer.

You may create an atmosphere that supports peak health and energy by partaking in activities that enhance your well-being.

Your energy and vigour are directly impacted by increasing your vibrational frequency. You might frequently feel worn out, lethargic, and unmotivated when your frequency is low. However, when your vibrational frequency rises, you get access to a reservoir of renewed vigour and energy. You can direct this extra energy into your career, relationships, and other pursuits, as well as into different areas of your life. You can discover that you have more endurance, concentration, and zeal when taking on chores and participating in physical activities. Regular movement and exercise become fun and energising, further enhancing your well-being.

Furthermore, increasing your vibrational frequency can help injuries and illnesses heal more quickly. When given the correct circumstances, the body has a remarkable ability to mend itself. By increasing your vibrational frequency, you foster a healing environment that quickens recovery time. Your body's balanced energy flow promotes cellular regeneration and repair, which aids in the healing of damaged tissues.

A faster healing process can also be facilitated by the optimistic outlook and emotional stability that come with a higher vibratory frequency. According to studies, people with an optimistic mindset frequently have better results from procedures, suffer fewer injuries, and recover from illnesses and accidents more quickly.

It's crucial to understand that increasing your vibrational frequency involves many different facets of your life. It entails making good lifestyle decisions for your physical body as well as working on your emotional and mental well-being. Your vibrational frequency can be increased by incorporating techniques like meditation, mindfulness, positive affirmations, and energy-healing therapies. Spending time in nature, surrounding oneself with uplifting connections, and participating in joyful hobbies can all help you achieve a higher vibratory level.

There are several advantages to increasing your vibrational frequency for your physical health and vigour. You lay the groundwork for optimal well-being by enhancing your immune system, raising your energy levels, and promoting quicker healing and recovery. Living a more active, joyful, and resilient life might result from adopting a holistic approach to health that takes into account the mind, body, and spirit.

Increased Mental Focus and Clarity

The ability to concentrate and think clearly are becoming more and more valuable skills in today's fast-paced, information-driven environment. Success in a variety of spheres of life, such as employment, education, and personal pursuits, depends on one's capacity for clear thought, concentration, and focus. The improvement of mental clarity and focus can be considerably aided by raising one's vibrational frequency. This article investigates the advantages of a higher vibrational frequency in connection to enhanced creativity and problem-solving abilities, expanded cognitive capacities and memory, and improved concentration and attention span.

Improved Memory and Cognitive Skills:

The functioning of the brain and cognitive capacities are positively impacted when a person raises their vibrational frequency. Increased cerebral activity and connectivity are linked to higher vibrational frequencies, which enhance overall brain function. This improvement appears in a variety of ways, including:

Learning Capacity and Information Processing: People with higher vibrational frequencies frequently have better learning and information-processing abilities. They are better able to assimilate, comprehend, and integrate new information, which results in a deeper comprehension of challenging ideas.

Higher vibrational frequencies have been associated with enhanced memory retention and recall. People with higher vibrational frequencies frequently have an easier time storing and retrieving knowledge in both short- and long-term memory.

Increased Vibrational Frequency: Increasing one's vibrational frequency might hasten brain processing. This implies that people can think and act more quickly, which can be especially useful in decision-making circumstances or when working on time-sensitive jobs.

Improved Problem-Solving and Creativity:

For innovation, adaptation, and success in a variety of fields, problem-solving abilities and creativity are essential. These cognitive capacities can be considerably improved by increasing one's vibrational frequency. This is how:

Higher vibratory frequencies allow the mind to be more open to broader viewpoints and unusual thought processes. This broader perspective enables people to approach issues from fresh perspectives, which produces ground-breaking ideas and discoveries.

Access to Intuitive Insights: People frequently experience enhanced intuition and inner direction when their vibratory frequency is elevated. This can result in creative "aha" moments when answers or ideas appear to come to you without effort. Such intuitive insights can be helpful in both creative and problem-solving endeavours.

Raising vibrational frequency assists people in letting go of mental obstacles and limiting beliefs that could impede their ability to be creative and solve problems. By letting go of these constraints, people are free to investigate novel concepts and avenues, which enhances creativity and improves problem-solving.

Greater Capacity for Concentration and Maintaining Focus:

Focus has grown more difficult to retain in today's world of distractions. Concentration and sustained focus can be greatly enhanced by increasing one's vibrational frequency. This is how it can be done:

Increased Present-Moment Awareness and Mindfulness: Higher vibrational frequencies encourage present-moment awareness and mindfulness. People who are more at the moment are better able to identify and control distractions, which helps them focus more intently on the task at hand.

Elevated vibrational frequencies are connected to a calmer mind, which lessens mental chatter and inner restlessness. People may maintain their composure and concentration on their duties without becoming absorbed by off-task thoughts thanks to this tranquillity.

Raising one's vibrational frequency can help one be more resilient and have greater mental fortitude. People with higher frequencies frequently find it simpler to maintain concentration and remain interested in projects for longer periods of time. They are more able to overcome obstacles and keep their focus when faced with problems.

Additionally, a higher vibrational frequency encourages innovation and problem-solving abilities. Higher vibrational persons can tackle difficulties with new insights and creative ideas by broadening their perspectives and thought patterns. A higher vibrational frequency can open up the door to intuitive insights, which can lead to innovative ideas and fresh approaches to challenging issues. People can unlock their creativity and venture into the unexplored territory by letting go of mental barriers and limiting beliefs.

Increased concentration and sustained focus on tasks are two benefits of increasing vibrational frequency. The capacity to remain focused and involved in the present moment is essential in a world full of distractions. A higher vibrational frequency encourages mindfulness and present-moment awareness, which makes it easier for people to spot and avoid distractions. People can maintain attention and prevent being distracted by unimportant ideas thanks to the decreased mental chatter and inner unrest brought on by a higher vibrational frequency.

One's mental resilience and endurance are improved by increasing vibrational frequency. It gives people the resilience and inner fortitude they need to overcome obstacles and keep their focus in the face of difficulty. People with this mental toughness can persevere through activities and projects, which boosts productivity and helps them reach their goals.

It is significant to remember that increasing one's vibrational frequency is an all-encompassing process involving several routines and practises. Vibrational frequency can be raised by partaking in practices like meditation, mindfulness exercises, regular physical activity, positive affirmations, and surrounding oneself with uplifting and positive influences. The above-mentioned cognitive benefits result from these practices' ability to align one's ideas, emotions, and behaviour with higher vibrations.

Raising one's vibrational frequency has major advantages for improved mental clarity and focus. People who have better cognitive skills and memories are able to learn more efficiently, remember knowledge, and think more rapidly. Individuals are more able to approach problems with new perspectives and creative solutions when they have improved creativity and problem-solving abilities. Increased productivity and the capacity to ignore distractions come from improved concentration and sustained attention to tasks. Raising one's vibratory frequency is a life-changing journey that includes a variety of behaviours and routines to harmonise one's mind, body, and spirit, ultimately resulting in a more successful and meaningful existence.

Enhanced Interactions

A vital component of human life is in relationships that are healthy and fulfilling. We gain a number of advantages that have a favourable effect on our interpersonal connections when we enhance our vibrational frequency. This essay examines three main advantages: improved interpersonal empathy and compassion, improved interpersonal communication and understanding, and the allure of wholesome and harmonious partnerships.

Increased empathy and compassion for others

Raising our vibratory frequency enables us to develop a more profound sense of empathy and compassion for others. We become more mindful of the interconnection of all beings as we synchronise with higher states of consciousness. Greater knowledge of the struggles, feelings, and experiences of others results from this awareness. We approach relationships with kindness, patience, and a sincere desire to help and uplift others around us when we have greater compassion and empathy.

By providing a secure environment for openness and emotional closeness, compassion and empathy promote stronger connections. We may respond with empathy and offer solace, certainty, and a sense of belonging when we actually comprehend and acknowledge the thoughts, feelings, and viewpoints of others. This degree of emotional intimacy promotes trust and builds ties, resulting in more satisfying and lasting partnerships.

Enhanced Understanding and Communication in Relationships

Our ability to communicate effectively and improve our capacity for understanding and being understood by others are both positively impacted by raising our vibrational frequency. We become more alert, present, and attentive in our interactions as our consciousness rises. More successful communication results from our ability to actively listen, empathise, and reply in an authentic manner when we are present.

We gain more emotional intelligence, which helps us recognise and control our own emotions and comprehend the emotions of others by increasing our vibrational frequency. The reduction of misunderstandings, disputes, and unneeded conflict in relationships is made possible by this emotional intelligence.

We also become more conscious of non-verbal clues, body language, and subtle nuances in communication as our vibrational frequency is raised. Because of our increased awareness, we can better understand signals and tailor our responses to meet the needs and intentions of others. It enables sensitive communication, which strengthens connection and understanding in our relationships.

Bringing About Harmonious and Positive Connections

The kind of relationships we bring into our life can be significantly changed by increasing our vibrational frequency. Our vibratory frequency attracts events and other people who are in tune with our energy. When we elevate our vibration, we produce uplifting, harmonious vibrations that draw other energies that are like ours.

Mutual respect, support, and progress are characteristics of relationships that are successful and harmonious. We are more likely to meet others who share our values, ambitions, and goals when our vibrational frequency is higher. These connections uplift us, encourage us, and support our general well-being.

Additionally, as we increase our vibrational frequency, we learn to be more selective in our dating. We acquire a sharpened intuition that enables us to identify poisonous or unhealthy dynamics and consciously choose to break them off. By exercising discernment, we can make sure that we devote our time and effort to connections that enrich and nurture us, thereby fostering a supportive and encouraging atmosphere.

Our relationships gain a lot by increasing our vibrational frequency. Deeper connections are fostered by greater compassion and empathy, and more fruitful encounters result from improved communication and understanding. By tuning into higher frequencies, we draw in uplifting and peaceful relationships that support our development and well-being.

As we keep raising our vibratory frequency, love, compassion, and understanding expand throughout the planet as a result. In the end, we help to create a more peaceful and integrated society by nourishing our connections through a higher vibrating state.

Growth and Awareness of the Spiritual

Beyond membership with a particular religion, spiritual development and awareness connect people with their inner selves, greater consciousness, and the divine. Through this journey, one can experience deep personal growth, inner tranquilly, and a better understanding of the world and its place in it. In this section, we'll look at how spiritual development and awareness help people to feel more connected to their higher selves or to divine consciousness, develop their spiritual wisdom and intuition, and develop a stronger sense of purpose and alignment with their life's mission.

Enhanced Relationship with the Divine or Higher Self

Developing a stronger relationship with one's higher self or divine consciousness, which can be thought of as the essence of our actual nature outside of the ego, is a common aspect of spiritual progress. Here we tap into a greater wisdom and universal truth that transcends the boundaries of the physical world. People can reach this deeper aspect of themselves and feel a profound sense of connection and interconnectedness with all of creation through practices like meditation, prayer, or contemplation.

People have a deeper sense of inner guidance and a wider perspective on life as their connection with their higher selves deepens. They develop a stronger intuition, which enables individuals to make decisions and choices that are in line with their authentic selves. People can find a source of unwavering love, knowledge, and support through this connection, which enables them to face their issues head-on and with grace.

Enhanced intuitive and spiritual insights

People frequently have deeper spiritual insights and sharper intuition when they start their spiritual growth journeys. The term "spiritual insights" describes the profound comprehension and knowledge that result from establishing a connection with the higher reaches of consciousness. People get fresh viewpoints on life, interpersonal relationships, and the nature of reality as a result of this increased awareness.

Deep truths about the interdependence of all things, the transience of material wealth, and the significance of compassion and love can be revealed via spiritual insights. These epiphanies frequently contradict accepted wisdom and present fresh perspectives and methods of being in the world.

Additionally, spiritual development strengthens intuition, which is the inner knowing or gut instinct that helps people make decisions that are in line with their highest benefit. When faced with uncertainty, intuition serves as a compass, offering direction and a sense of confidence. It enables people to access their inner wisdom and take actions that are consistent with who they truly are, which promotes personal development and results in more satisfying experiences.

Enhanced Purpose and Alignment with One's Life Path

Increased feelings of purpose and congruence with one's life path are two of the most powerful outcomes of spiritual development and awareness. As people progress in their spiritual development, they start to recognise their own abilities, skills, and passions. Through self-discovery, one gains a deeper understanding of their life's purpose and a sense of fulfilment that transcends material success or worldly accomplishments.

Spiritual development enables people to live more authentically and meaningfully by enabling them to align their actions, values, and ambitions with their soul's purpose. It offers advice on how to live in accordance with one's values and objectives and clarifies what really matters. As a result of feeling as though they are living a life with meaning and making a positive difference in the world, people who are in harmony have a great sense of joy, fulfilment, and inner peace.

Spiritual development and awakening are transformative journeys that help people to connect more deeply with their higher selves or divine consciousness, develop their spiritual intuition and insights, and feel more purposeful and in accordance with their life's purpose. Individuals can go on this path and experience significant personal growth, inner calm, and a better knowledge of their place in the world through practices, including meditation, contemplation, and self-reflection. People can build a greater feeling of meaning and fulfilment in their life by fostering these components of spiritual growth, which will benefit both their own well-being and communal awareness.

Possibility and Abundance

The ideas of manifestation and abundance are interrelated and have attracted a lot of attention lately. The principle of manifestation holds that our thoughts, beliefs, and energy have the power to affect reality and produce the results we want. A higher state of consciousness that enables us to align with abundance and draw what we want into our life is accessed when we elevate our vibratory frequency. The tremendous effects of raising one's vibrational frequency on manifestation and abundance will be discussed in this section.

Improved capacity to attract and bring about desired results

Raising our vibratory frequency allows us to more fully grasp the power of manifestation and provides a doorway to the world of possibilities. Our ideas, feelings, beliefs, and general energy all affect the vibrational frequency of our bodies. We elevate our vibration and produce a magnetic field that pulls in other frequencies when we actively choose to nurture positive ideas, emotions, and beliefs.

We can stay in a high vibratory state and go closer to our goals and ambitions. As we naturally draw others, situations, and chances that support our objectives and aspirations, we start to see a change in our reality. Our greater capacity to bring about desired outcomes becomes clear, whether it be manifesting a rewarding profession, love relationships, better health, or financial wealth.

Enhanced coincidences and opportunities

Synchronicities are significant coincidences that take place in our lives and show that we are in harmony with the universe's natural flow. These synchronicities happen more frequently and clearly when we increase our vibratory frequency because we are more tuned in to them.

The cosmos works together to deliver us chances and experiences that are in line with our desires when we align ourselves with a higher vibratory level. We might come upon helpful resources, the right people at the right moment, or unanticipated help from unanticipated places.

Additionally, increasing our vibrational frequency enables us to see chances that we might have previously missed. Our enhanced intuition and increased awareness help us spot these chances and take advantage of them, which results in more growth and abundance in our life.

In 1982 I was traveling from New England to Texas pulling a small uhaul trailer behind a '79 corolla, I experienced directly a happy coincidence that acted as one of the universe's gentle nudges, pointing us in the direction of the fulfilment of our aspirations.

I had missed my exit, and could not back up the car with trailer on the interstate. It was in the wee hours of the morning, no other traffic on the road and I was in an unfamiliar location. The grassy area between the shoulder of the interstate where I was, and the off ramp, where I wanted to be, was only about 15 feet. In my young, unexperienced mind, I thought I could just drove over the grass and be back on track in a minute. As I drove across the small median, I discovered that the grass had hidden a ditch, where I now found myself homelessly stuck. I allowed my emotions to take over for a minute, then took some deep breaths to calm and balance myself. It was then that I looked up into my rearview mirror and saw headlights in a distance.

As the headlights got closer, they started to slow down, then came to a complete stop on the shoulder of the road behind me.

> Coincidence #1- the truck was a tow truck
> Coincidence #2- the driver had a daughter the same age as I, also expecting, also in the military.

He pulled my car out of the ditch, leaving me on the off ramp, in the direction I needed to be, and asked me to pay it forward.

The experience left an imprint that has prompted years of seeking to understand the energy of emotion and how it plays into our reality.

Willingness to receive abundance in all aspects of life

We develop an abundant attitude and make ourselves more receptive to obtaining abundance in all spheres of our lives when we raise our vibratory frequency. This encompasses a variety of abundances, such as material, psychological, and spiritual.

Raising our vibratory frequency aids us in letting go of money-related limiting patterns and beliefs. In order to create experiences and have a positive impact, we learn to have a positive relationship with money. As our vibrational frequency increases, we draw in chances for success, prosperity, and progress in all spheres of life.

The emotions of happiness, love, gratitude, and contentment are all included in emotional abundance. Raising our vibrational frequency improves our emotional health and makes it easier for us to feel and give off happy feelings. We develop a greater sense of gratitude for the present moment and experience more delight in our daily lives. As a result, we draw more positive encounters and fulfilling connections into our lives.

A strong relationship with our higher selves or divine consciousness is necessary for spiritual abundance. We can experience significant spiritual growth, inner serenity, and a feeling of direction by increasing our vibrational frequency. As we go closer to following our spiritual path, (alignment with our higher purpose) we develop greater clarity and understanding of the course of our lives.

It's crucial to remember that increasing our vibratory frequency and attracting riches are about more than just accumulating wealth. It is about living a life of integrity and fulfilment, expressing our special gifts, and being in alignment with our authentic selves.

Our capacity to manifest and draw riches changes when we raise our vibrational frequency. By actively making positive decisions regarding our ideas, feelings, and beliefs, we connect to the energy of abundance and widen our range of options. We develop our ability to materialise the results we want, observe how opportunities and synchronicities present themselves, and foster abundance throughout our lives. Raising our vibratory frequency and embracing the power of manifestation and abundance give us the ability to conciously build the life we truly want.

Positive Environmental Effects

An increase in vibrational frequency has a cascading effect on everyone's consciousness.

Raising one's vibrational frequency offers benefits that go beyond just improving one's own health; it also has the ability to have a positive effect on the environment. The energetic condition of an individual or a collective consciousness is referred to as vibrational frequency, and when it is high, it has the power to affect people's ideas, feelings, and behaviours. The ripple effect of this shift can spread to the collective consciousness as individuals try to raise their vibrational frequencies, leading to an increase in awareness and care for the environment.

People who increase their vibratory frequency become more aware of the connectivity of all living things and grow to feel a sense of oneness with the natural world. This increased awareness encourages a deeper comprehension of how their actions affect the environment. People begin to understand that their actions and decisions have the potential to either negatively impact the state of the world or pave the way for a more sustainable future.

Greater sensitivity to and regard for the environment

The development of a greater sense of care and respect for the environment is one of the key advantages of raising one's vibrational frequency. High Vibe people start to regard the Earth as a living being deserving of love, protection, and preservation as they start to align with their life's purpose. This change in perspective leads to practical actions that put the welfare of the earth first.

People with higher vibrational frequencies frequently incorporate sustainable habits into their daily lives. They start to pay attention to their consumption habits, choosing eco-friendly goods, cutting back on waste, and engaging in responsible resource management. People could decide to recycle, support local and organic agriculture, use renewable energy sources, or take an active role in conservation initiatives.

Additionally, a high vibrational frequency encourages a strong bond with nature. People are spending more time outside, enjoying parks, forests, and beaches, among other natural settings. A deep appreciation for the beauty and wealth of the Earth is fostered by this communion with nature, which bolsters the desire to preserve it. To actively contribute to environmental preservation, people can take part in projects like planting trees, cleaning up beaches, or wildlife protection.

Contribution to fostering a world that is more peaceful and sustainable

Increased environmental awareness is a result of raising vibrational frequency, which also makes the planet more peaceful and sustainable. The collective consciousness changes as more people choose a higher vibratory state, leading to a shift towards more sustainable practices and international collaboration.

People begin to understand the value of cooperation and unification to confront environmental concerns when the collective consciousness is influenced by raised vibrational frequencies. They are aware that collaborating for the greater good transcends national boundaries, partisan differences, and individual interests. This harmony provides the path for global cooperation on environmental problems, including pollution, deforestation, and climate change.

Higher vibrational frequencies also encourage the creation and adoption of ground-breaking environmental solutions. People with higher levels of consciousness are more receptive to novel concepts, innovations, and strategies that can lessen the negative effects of human activity on the environment. This mentality change promotes scholarly inquiry, technology development, and the adoption of sustainable practices across a range of sectors.

Furthermore, a change in attitudes and priorities is necessary for a peaceful and sustainable society. People are prompted to reconsider their definitions of success and happiness when the vibrational frequency rises. A focus on well-being, meaningful connections, and the preservation of the planet for future generations takes the place of materialistic pursuits. A culture of conscious consumerism is fostered by this paradigm shift, in which people give greater weight to the ecological and social consequences of their decisions than to their financial gain.

Raising one's vibrational frequency has a good effect on the environment in addition to one's own health. People gain a higher feeling of concern and respect for the environment by expanding their consciousness and establishing a closer connection with nature. This mentality change results in a dedication to environmental preservation and sustainable lifestyle choices.

Furthermore, by encouraging international cooperation, encouraging creative solutions, and pushing a change in values towards conscious consumption, the ripple effect of raised vibrational frequencies in the collective consciousness leads to the development of a more peaceful and sustainable society. In the end, the favourable effects on the environment brought about by increasing vibrational frequency may significantly contribute to assuring a prosperous future for the planet and all of its inhabitants.

Chapter 4: What is the connection between thoughts, behaviors, and vibrations?

Vibrations and actions?

The interactions of thoughts, actions, and vibrations that make up the human experience are intricate. These three factors interact with one another in complex ways, profoundly impacting and forming one another. Knowing how thoughts, actions, and vibrations interact can help us better understand our mental, emotional, and even physical health.

Everything in the cosmos is fundamentally made of energy. Even thoughts have energy. Our minds produce electromagnetic waves that have specific frequencies or vibrations while we think. Beyond the confines of our physical bodies, these vibrations produce an energy field that interacts with the environment.

Similar to how our actions are not independent of this dynamic dance. The thoughts that come before our acts frequently shape them. Our perceptions, ideas, and attitudes are shaped by our thoughts, and these, in turn, affect our choices and behaviors. Therefore, our actions and energy output can be greatly influenced by the quality of our thoughts.

In this sense, the term "vibrations" refers to the energetic frequency at which humans function. Our ideas and actions cause vibrations that may be detected energetically, just as different musical notes have different frequencies. These vibrations, which indicate either favourable or unfavourable states of being, can have a wide variety of frequencies.

Higher vibrations are sent by ideas that are positive, such as love, gratitude, and joy. They are in tune with the vibrations of harmony, abundance, and well-being. Negative emotions like fear, rage, and resentment, on the other hand, produce lower vibrations. These vibrations match those that are linked to lack, discord, and illness.

Through the perspective of the Law of Attraction, it is possible to better comprehend how thoughts, actions, and vibrations are connected. This universal law states that opposites attract. When we continually think and act positively, positive energy and events are drawn into our lives. On the other hand, unfavourable feelings and actions can draw unfavourable energies and experiences.

In this interaction, conscious awareness is essential. Being aware of our thoughts and actions gives us the ability to change our vibrational frequencies on purpose. We can notice our thoughts and behaviours, spot patterns, and make deliberate decisions to match with higher vibratory states by using the tools of mindfulness and self-reflection.

It's critical to understand that thoughts, actions, and vibrations are connected in a feedback loop. Our vibrations are influenced by our behaviors, which in turn are influenced by our ideas. Similar to how our ideas and actions can be reinforced by our vibrations, this can result in a never-ending cycle of either positive or negative energy.

This interconnectivity has effects that go beyond the metaphysical sphere. Positive attitudes and actions can actually have a noticeable impact on our mental, emotional, and physical health, according to research in the field of psycho-neuro-immunology. We can experience more resilience, better relationships, and better general health by cultivating positive ideas, practising healthy behaviors, and emitting higher vibrational frequencies.

Applications for daily use become possible if we comprehend the link between ideas, actions, and vibrations. We can raise our vibrational frequencies and create positive thoughts and behaviors by using strategies like affirmations, journaling, meditation, visualisation, gratitude exercises, and acts of kindess. Making these routines a part of our lives helps us maintain higher vibratory states and attract great events. The key is consistency and intention.

Exactly What Thoughts Are

Our daily lives are impacted by our thoughts, which shape how we see and interact with the environment. They influence our feelings, actions, and general well-being. In order to acquire insight into the workings of our brains and utilise their ability to effect positive change, it is necessary to comprehend the nature of thoughts. In this chapter, we'll look at what thoughts are, what makes them tick, how they affect our perception, experience, and more. We'll also discuss the importance of thinking positively vs. negatively and how that affects our life.

Thoughts' definition and characteristics

The mental processes that produces ideas, attitudes, and beliefs are known as thoughts. They represent the internal discourse that permeates our minds on a constant basis, generating both conscious and unconscious mental activity. Our cognitive processes, which include perception, memory, attention, and reasoning, produce thoughts.

Volatility: Thoughts are erratic and constantly shifting. They arrive and vanish swiftly, frequently flowing mindlessly from one to the next. Thoughts become dynamic and continually change as a result of this volatility.

Subjectivity: Thoughts are deeply individualised and subjective. Our values, experiences, and beliefs all have an impact on them, forming our particular worldview. One person's perspective on a certain circumstance may be very different from another person's perspective on the same issue.

Thoughts are creative in their nature. They have the ability to spark innovation, find solutions to issues, and produce fresh ideas. We are able to imagine possibilities, think abstractly, and exercise critical thought because of our capacity for creative thought.

Thoughts can be classified as being either positive or negative, helpful or harmful, empowering or limiting. This dualism results from the interaction of our conscious and subconscious minds as well as external factors like cultural indoctrination and societal conventions.

The influence of thoughts on perception and experience:

Our thoughts have a significant impact on how we experience and view the world. They serve as filters through which we interpret relationships, circumstances, and occurrences. The following examples demonstrate how our perception and experience are influenced by our thoughts:

Cognitive biases, which are regular patterns of judgmental deviance from objectivity or reason, can have an impact on thoughts. These biases can cause us to see and interpret information in a flawed way, which can have an impact on our ability to make decisions and comprehend the world as a whole.

Emotional control: Thoughts and emotions are intricately linked. Emotional responses can be sparked by thoughts, and thoughts, in turn, can be influenced by emotions. We can control and manage our emotions by intentionally forming our thoughts, which fosters emotional resilience and well-being.

Interpretation of Experiences: Our interpretation of experiences is framed by our thoughts, which also determine whether we see them as rewarding or challenging, positive or negative. Depending on our thinking, the same incident might be understood in a variety of ways, leading to various emotional and behavioral reactions.

Self-Image and Self-Efficacy: Important components of our psychological well-being, self-image and self-efficacy are influenced by our thoughts. A healthy self-perception, increased self-confidence, and improved self-belief can all be cultivated by thinking positively. On the other hand, negative thoughts can result in insecurity, a low sense of self-worth, and a lessened sense of effectiveness.

The Influence of Both Positive and Negative Thoughts

Our lives are greatly influenced by our thoughts, both positive and negative, which shape our experiences, relationships, and general well-being. The potential of positive thinking to foster optimism, toughness, and a proactive mindset is what gives it its strength. Negative thinking, on the other side, can cause tension, anxiety, and a pessimistic perspective. What is their importance?

Positive Thoughts

Positive thinking creates optimism, which enables us to approach problems with a solution-focused attitude. Optimism and resilience. It increases resiliency, assisting us in overcoming obstacles and disappointments.

Emotional Well-Being: Positive emotions are produced by thinking positively, which enhances one's mental and emotional health. They can ease sadness, anxiety, and stress, leading to a more contented and balanced life.

Relationships: Thinking positively affects how we interact with others. It encourages compassion, empathy, and kindness, which improves the calibre of our interactions.

Negative Thoughts

Pessimism and Self-Fulfilling Prophecy: Imposter Syndrome, or worrying about one's shortcomings and failings is a common result of negative thinking. This way of thinking can cause unfavourable outcomes to continue and prevent human development.

Emotional Distress: Negative emotions are fueled by negative ideas, which raise tension, worry, and dissatisfaction levels. They may reduce one's quality of life and general well-being.

Relationship Impact: Because it can result in more criticism, cynicism, and disagreements, negative thinking can put relationships under stress. It could put up obstacles to clear communication and comprehension.

Our perspectives, experiences, and general well-being are all shaped by the thoughts we have. For personal development and self-awareness, it is essential to understand their nature, traits, and functions in our life. The difference between how we think positively and negatively affects our mental, emotional, and social well-being, emphasising the value of developing positive thought patterns. We may use the transforming power of our brains to create a more meaningful and joyful experience of life by becoming aware of our ideas and intentionally selecting good viewpoints.

Human Behavior and Its Influence

Our lives are significantly shaped by our behaviors, which also have an impact on our general well-being. They interact dynamically with our thoughts and vibrations, changing how we perceive the world and how we experience it. We will go into the knowledge of behaviors, their connection to thoughts, and their effect on our vibrations in this section. We'll also look at how recognising trends and behaviors, understanding your triggers, may keep our overall vibration positive.

Understanding actions and how they relate to thinking

The actions and conduct we engage in on a daily basis are known as behaviors. They are an expression of our feelings, thoughts, and emotions on the outside. Our decisions are influenced by our thoughts, which in turn shape our behaviors. As a result, there is a constant feedback loop between our actions and ideas.

Link Between Thought and Behavior:

Our behaviors are built upon our thoughts. Poor ideas can result in poor behaviors, whereas happy thoughts can cause positive behaviors. For instance, someone is more likely to take the initiative and behave in ways that support their goals if they believe they can achieve them.

Loop of Behavior-Thought Feedback

In addition to being the result of thoughts, behaviours also have the capacity to influence and reinforce our mental patterns. Repeatedly carrying out certain behaviours can reinforce related cognitive patterns, resulting in a feedback loop. For instance, performing deeds of kindness repeatedly can foster a positive outlook and strengthen faith in people.

Examining how actions affect vibrations and thoughts

Our actions have a significant impact on our thoughts and vibrations, which in turn affects how we feel overall and the experiences we attract.

Alignment of Behaviour and Thoughts:

Congruence and a sense of sincerity are felt when our actions match our thoughts and beliefs. This connection improves our mental attitude and emotional health. Contrarily, acting in ways that go against our beliefs might result in cognitive dissonance, which causes internal conflict and has a detrimental impact on our thoughts.

Behaviour and the Impact of Vibration:

Every action produces a vibration that modifies our body's total energy frequency. Higher vibrations are emitted by positive behaviors like gratitude, compassion, and generosity, which attract other happy experiences that are similar to them. On the other hand, bad behaviors like jealousy, wrath, or dishonesty reduce our vibratory frequency, which attracts unfavourable situations.

Identifying trends and routines that influence our overall vibration:

It is crucial to recognise patterns and habits that can be harmful to our well-being and seek to cultivate good alternatives if we want to keep our overall vibration positive.

Self-Awareness and Reflection:

Self-awareness is essential for identifying behavioural patterns that can affect our thoughts and vibrations. Regular self-reflection enables us to view our behaviour objectively, spot any troubling trends, and comprehend the underlying causes of those behaviors.

Changing Adverse Patterns:

Conscious attempts can be made to break free from destructive patterns and habits after they have been acknowledged. This entails swapping out unfavourable behaviours for constructive ones that correspond to our desired ideas and vibrations. Implementing time-management strategies and encouraging discipline, for instance, can assist in breaking a tendency to procrastinate.

Developing Good Habits:

Positive habits that are intentionally developed can have a tremendous impact on our overall vibration. Daily mental and behavioural alignment with higher vibratory frequencies can be reinforced by practising mindfulness, gratitude, and self-care.

Our experiences and general well-being are shaped by our behaviours, which are fundamental to our thoughts and vibrations. Knowing the link between our actions, thoughts, and vibrations enables us to actively select behaviors that support the outcomes we want. We can maintain a high vibrational frequency and draw experiences that are in line with our highest objectives by recognising negative patterns and developing positive habits.

Exploring the Concept of Vibrations

Understanding vibrations and how they relate to feelings and actions

Our reality is largely shaped by vibrations, which are an essential component of our life. Everything in the universe, from the smallest subatomic particles to the greatest celestial entities, is fundamentally vibrating. The world around us is created and influenced by these vibrations, which can be thought of as energy waves.

We discover that our ideas and emotions produce their own distinctive frequencies when we investigate the relationship between vibrations, thoughts, and behaviours. Higher frequencies are produced by elevating and uplifting thoughts, whereas lower frequencies are produced by restricting and negative thinking. These frequencies have the power to affect how we act and how happy we feel in general.

Our thoughts serve as a catalyst, setting off a series of events that have an impact on our emotions, beliefs, and, ultimately, our actions. For instance, if we frequently think and believe things like "I'm not good enough" or "I always fail," these vibrations reverberate inside of us and can show up as self-destructive behaviors or a lack of confidence. On the other side, nurturing optimistic and energising thoughts can result in actions that support achievement and personal development.

Acquiring knowledge of the vibrational frequency spectrum

From low to high frequencies, the idea of vibrational frequency spans a spectrum. Denser and slower vibrations are found at the lower end of the spectrum, while lighter and faster vibrations are found at the higher end. It's crucial to remember that no frequency is fundamentally good or evil; instead, they all have different functions and experiences.

Negative emotions like fear, rage, guilt, and others are frequently linked to low-frequency vibrations. These frequencies can take the form of self-destructive habits, constrained viewpoints, and a sense of isolation from the outside world. We can go towards higher frequencies by partaking in vibration-raising activities like gratitude practice, meditation, or enjoyable hobbies.

On the other side, good feelings such as love, joy, and serenity are included in high-frequency vibrations. These vibrations enable us to live with clarity, direction, and fulfilment because they are in alignment with our actual identity. As like attracts like, we draw pleasant experiences and people into our lives when we resonate at higher frequencies.

Vibrations' part in the Law of Attraction

According to the Law of Attraction, which was made well-known by the book "The Secret," opposites attract. It implies that we attract situations into our lives that is consistent with the vibrations we create through our thoughts and emotions. In other words, the energy we emit into the universe returns to us in different ways.

The Law of Attraction states that when we continually think and feel positively, we align with higher vibrations and draw favourable circumstances and opportunities to ourselves. On the other hand, when we focus on negative feelings and thoughts, we align with lower vibrations and draw more of the same into our lives.

Aligning our thoughts, feelings, and vibrations with the results we want is crucial if we want to fully utilise the Law of Attraction. This entails developing an optimistic outlook, engaging in acts of gratitude, visualising our objectives, and acting on inspiration. We can improve our capacity for manifesting our desires and forging a more fulfilling reality by intentionally boosting our vibration and upholding a positive frame of mind.

It's important to remember that the Law of Attraction does not provide a quick fix for manifestation; rather, it calls for persistent effort, self-awareness, and a strong conviction in the power of vibrations. It is a tool that, when used correctly, may assist us in altering our vision, drawing in advantageous circumstances, and ultimately building a life that is consistent with our deepest wishes.

Our existence depends on vibrations because they link our ideas, actions, and experiences. We can actively attempt to raise our frequency and align ourselves with favourable results by comprehending the nature of vibrations and their impact on our life. A framework for using vibrations to manifest our wishes and produce a happier, more fulfilling reality is provided by the Law of Attraction. We can become conscious makers of our own experiences and live in accordance with our fullest potential by harnessing the power of our ideas and emotions.

The interaction of vibrations, actions, and thoughts

The deep and interesting interplay that exists between thoughts, actions, and vibrations has a significant impact on how we conduct our daily lives. Our ideas influence our actions, and those actions have a significant influence on our vibrations. Knowing how these factors interact can provide us with important insights into how to foster good and congruent experiences. This section will study the relationship between how thoughts affect behaviors and how behaviours affect thoughts, as well as the influence of vibrations on both. We will also look at case studies and instances that highlight the relationship.

How actions are influenced by thoughts, and vice versa

Behaviours are shaped by thoughts:

Our actions and behaviours are built on the foundation of our thinking. Our behaviors are greatly influenced by how we view the world, the ideas we have, and the internal dialogue we have. While negative ideas can result in self-destructive or harmful behaviours, good thoughts frequently lead to positive acts. For instance, if a person continually feels unworthy, they may engage in self-defeating behaviours like isolating themselves or refusing new possibilities.

Actions that support thoughts:

Additionally, actions might support our thoughts and beliefs. We reinforce a specific cognitive pattern when we repeatedly engage in a particular behavior. For instance, if a person frequently avoids speaking events because they believe they are bad at public speaking, their avoidance behavior reinforces that belief. It becomes harder to break out from a negative mind habit as a result of this reinforcement. I like to think of it as repetitious thoughts create beliefs. Beliefs influence emotions, behaviors and actions.

CBT: Cognitive behavioural therapy

Understanding how ideas and behaviors interact creates possibilities for constructive change. The main goal of cognitive-behavioral approaches is to recognise negative beliefs, challenge them, and then replace them with more powerful and productive ones. We may change our behaviors to be more constructive by intentionally changing our ideas, which will ultimately affect our vibrations.

Investigating how vibrations affect attitudes and actions

Recognising vibrations:

Every person and thing in the cosmos emits some form of energetic frequency or resonance, which is referred to as vibrations. Our thoughts, feelings, and behaviors are vibrations, just like everything else in the universe. These vibrations have a magnetic nature that draws events and situations to themselves that match their frequency. Consequently, our vibrations have a big impact on how we think and act.

Harmonic alignment:

When our vibrations are in harmony with positivity, gratitude, and love, those qualities frequently manifest in our thoughts and deeds. Positive thoughts, acts of kindness, and behaviors that are advantageous to both ourselves and others are more likely to occur. On the other hand, when negativity, fear, or anger rule our vibrations, our thoughts and actions frequently reflect those lower frequencies.

Principle of Attraction:

According to the Law of Attraction, we draw into our lives events that match the vibrations we are sending out. Optimistic outcomes are attracted to us when we regularly think of empowering and optimistic ideas and link our actions with those thoughts. On the other hand, if our attitudes and actions are negative, our vibration will match that negativity, which will attract negative events.

Examples and case studies demonstrating the connection

Case Study: Mary's Development

Mary, a young professional, frequently questioned her skills and thought she would never succeed. Her views inspired self-destructive actions, such as putting off tasks and avoiding obstacles. She consequently suffered difficulties and lost possibilities. Mary discovered the link between her thoughts, behaviors, and vibrations via personal development work. She started saying encouraging things to herself, confronting her unfavourable thoughts, and stepping a little bit outside her comfort zone. Gradually, she started to think more positively and act in ways that were successful. Her vibration changed as a result, and she began to draw in new chances, which helped her experience tremendous career growth.

Example: The impact of appreciation:

A strong emotion and action that raises vibrations is gratitude. By recognising and appreciating the gifts in our lives, we may consciously cultivate thankfulness. When we do this, our thoughts become more upbeat, and our actions match with deeds of kindness and generosity. This raised vibration enhances connections, draws more fulfilling experiences, and improves general well-being.

Example: Emotional control and mindfulness

By using mindfulness techniques, we can examine our thoughts and feelings without passing judgement. We can recognise unfavorable or restricting ideas that motivate particular behaviours by becoming more conscious of our cognitive processes. We can learn to control our emotions by practising mindfulness and making conscious decisions to think and act in ways that support higher vibrations.

A dynamic and significant part of our existence is the interaction between our ideas, actions, and vibrations. A continual feedback loop results when thoughts are reinforced by behaviours. Our ideas, behaviours, and vibrations all have an effect on the events that resonate with our energetic frequency. Understanding and utilising this interaction will enable us to consciously control our thoughts, actions, and vibrations, ultimately leading to a happier and more fulfilled life.

Aligning Thoughts, Behaviours, and Vibrations: Techniques

Achieving personal growth, pleasure, and success requires alignment between thoughts, behaviors, and vibrations. When these three facets work together harmoniously, they provide a potent synergy that has the capacity to alter our lives. This article will examine three efficient approaches for bringing thoughts, actions, and vibrations into harmony: practises for mindfulness and awareness, cognitive-behavioural methods for thinking to restructure, and vibrational alignment and energy healing treatments.

Practises of Mindfulness and Awareness

Practises of mindfulness and awareness are crucial tools for bringing thoughts, behaviours, and vibrations into harmony. By practising present-moment awareness, we may more clearly see our thoughts and actions and make deliberate decisions to change our vibration.

Meditation: Regular meditation practice enables us to objectively observe our thoughts and feelings. Through meditation, we become more conscious of our thinking processes and acquire the ability to disengage from unfavourable or constricting thoughts. By doing this, we can better connect our ideas with empowering and positive ideals.

Deep, mindful breathing helps to relax the mind and pulls us into the present moment. We might choose to disconnect from unfavorable ideas by concentrating on our breath and instead directing it towards the good things in life. A more favorable vibrational state is encouraged by this practice.

Practise gratitude: Being grateful raises our vibratory frequency. We change our emphasis from scarcity to abundance by intentionally identifying and appreciating the blessings in our lives. A regular practice of thankfulness connects our thoughts, actions, and vibrations with the positive, inviting more favorable events.

Cognitive-Behavioural Strategies for Restructuring Thoughts

The use of cognitive-behavioural approaches can help us reorganise our ideas so that they correspond to the desired vibrations and behaviors. We may change our thought patterns and have a positive knock-on effect on our behaviours and vibrations by questioning and replacing negative or restricting beliefs.

Reframing negative or distorted beliefs is the goal of the cognitive reframing approach. We can change our negative beliefs into more empowering ones by weighing the evidence for and against them. Through the process of reframing, we can connect our beliefs with positive actions and higher vibrations.

Positive sentences that we frequently repeat to ourselves are called affirmations. We may rewire our subconscious minds by deliberately selecting affirmations that represent our ideal ideas, behaviours, and vibrations. By influencing our actions and attracting like-minded vibrations, affirmations assist us in connecting our thoughts with the world we want to create.

Visualisation: Visualisation entails constructing precise mental representations of our desired results. We match our ideas with those sensations by vividly visualising ourselves, carrying out constructive behaviours and experiencing desired vibrations. This connection inspires and directs our actions, accelerating the appearance of the world we want.

Methods of vibrational alignment and energy healing

Balancing and harmonising our energetic and vibrational frequencies is the main goal of energy healing and vibrational alignment techniques. Aligned thoughts and actions are the outcomes of these strategies' assistance in clearing obstructions, releasing bad energy, and raising our total vibratory level.

Reiki: Reiki is a therapeutic technique that encourages harmony and balance in the body and mind by utilising the universal life force energy. Practitioners can achieve a higher vibratory level by clearing energetic barriers through the channelling and direction of this energy. Reiki encourages inner healing and constructive transformation, which balances our ideas, behaviors, and vibrations.

Sound therapy: To encourage healing and alignment, sound therapy uses a range of precise frequencies and vibrations. Vibrations produced by instruments like singing bowls, tuning forks, or chanting resonant with various areas of our body and energy field. We can clear energetic blocks and harmonise our ideas, actions, and general vibratory frequency by experiencing these frequencies.

Crystal healing: Because each crystal has a different vibrational frequency, it can help us to align our thoughts, behaviours, and vibrations. We may amp up good vibrations and let go of bad ones by employing particular crystals because each crystal has unique qualities and energy. The alignment process is supported by crystal healing practises, including wearing crystals, meditating with them, or incorporating them into our surroundings.

A transforming process, aligning our thoughts, deeds, and vibrations, demands intentional effort and repetition. This alignment can be facilitated with the help of cognitive-behavioral strategies, mindfulness and awareness skills, and energy-healing approaches. We can develop a harmonious relationship between our ideas, actions, and vibrations by continuously using these approaches, which will promote personal development, fulfilment, and the realisation of our goals.

The Connection and Manifestation

The process of making our goals and aspirations come true is known as manifestation. As people look for ways to design the life they actually want, this idea has attracted a lot of attention recently. The relationship between thoughts, actions, and vibrations is essential to the manifestation process. Individuals can overcome challenges and maintain alignment for effective manifestation by comprehending this relationship and learning practical ways to utilise it.

The Function of Vibrations, Behaviors, and Thoughts in Manifestation:

Thoughts are the building blocks of manifestation. They have the ability to influence our thoughts, perceptions, and behavior. Consistently thinking of ideas that are in line with our desires causes us to vibrate at a frequency that draws chances and experiences that match.

Our actions are the outward manifestations of our thinking. They control how we behave and engage with the environment. By matching our actions to our desired manifestations, we strengthen our intentions and provide the universe with a clear indication of what we really want.

Everything in the universe emits vibrations since everything is made of energy. These vibrations can be strong or weak, favourable or unfavourable. We produce a high-frequency vibration that attracts to us the experiences and situations that resonate with that frequency when our thoughts and actions are in line with our desired manifestations

Using the Connection to Manifest Desires: Useful Advice

Identify and Clearly State Your Desires: Give your desires some thought. Think about what you want to materialise, and be clear and precise. This clarity aids in concentrating your thoughts, actions, and vibrations in the direction of your intended result.

Utilise affirmations that are favourable and visualisation strategies to strengthen your goals. While visualisation entails fervently imagining yourself already experiencing your desires, affirmations are positive remarks that reflect the reality you desire. Through these techniques, you can direct your thoughts and vibrations in the direction of the manifestations you want.

Take Inspired Action: Manifestation involves action as well as good thinking. Take motivated action that supports your goals. Your goals should be broken down into manageable milestones that you continually work towards achieving. Every action you take builds momentum and solidifies your faith in the manifestation process.

Develop a mindset of thankfulness and appreciation for the things you already have. Having gratitude increases your vibrational frequency, which invites more gifts into your life. Make it a habit to thank God every day for the manifestations in your life, both those you have already experienced and those still to come.

For successful manifestation, overcoming obstacles and keeping alignment is essential.

Identify and release any limiting thoughts that might be preventing you from manifesting your goals. Your confidence and faith in your capacity to manifest are undermined by limiting beliefs, which are ingrained thought patterns. Change them for empowering ideas that help you achieve your goals.

Self-reflection and self-awareness exercises can help you identify any unfavourable thought patterns or self-destructive behaviours that might be impeding your manifestations. Meditation and mindfulness are potent techniques that increase self-awareness and encourage alignment.

Trust the cosmos and Give Up Control: The process of manifesting is one in which you collaborate with the cosmos. Have faith that the universe has your back and is at work to make your dreams come true. Give up trying to manage everything, and let the cosmos bring about the manifestations in its own divine time.

Patience and Persistence: The process of manifestation is not always quick. It necessitates endurance and perseverance. Continue to connect your thoughts, actions, and vibrations with your intended result and have faith that your desires are coming true. Even in the face of obstacles or setbacks, remain devoted to your manifestations.

The relationship between thoughts, actions, and vibrations is at the heart of the potent process of manifestation. People can use this connection to their advantage by comprehending the function of each component and putting helpful advice into practice. The keys to successful manifestation are overcoming challenges and keeping alignment. Accept the ability you possess to consciously create the life you want, and watch as the universe answers to your intentions through the manifestations you desire.

Chapter 5: Brain and Emotions

Knowledge of the Olfactory Bulb

The Olfactory Bulb's Structure and Function

Placement and Design of the Olfactory Bulb

The crucial brain component that processes odor information is known as the olfactory bulb. It is located in the forebrain, specifically in the olfactory system at the base of the brain. The olfactory bulb is a tiny, oval-shaped organ with a normal length of a few centimetres. The olfactory nerve connects it to the olfactory epithelium, which is situated above the nasal cavity.

The Relationship Between Olfactory Receptor Neurons and the Olfactory Bulb

In order for the olfactory bulb to detect and transmit odor information, the olfactory receptor neurons (ORNs) are essential. Within the olfactory epithelium, which lines the nasal cavity, are these specialised neurons. The odorant receptors on the cilia of the olfactory receptor neurons allow them to recognise various odour compounds in the environment. An odor causes a signal that travels through the olfactory nerve fibres and eventually reaches the olfactory bulb when it attaches to a particular receptor.

The olfactory nerve, made up of the olfactory nerve fibres, is a bundle that transmits sensory data from the olfactory receptor neurons to the olfactory bulb. In particular areas of the olfactory bulb known as glomeruli, the olfactory nerve fibres come to an end.

Processing of Odor Information in the Olfactory Bulb

The olfactory bulb processes the odor information in great detail after it arrives. A crucial part of this process is played by the glomeruli in the olfactory bulb. A spatial map of the activation patterns of odorants is produced by the input that each glomerulus receives from a particular class of olfactory receptor neurons.

The transmission of information occurs within the glomeruli at the synapses between the olfactory nerve fibres and the dendrites of the mitral cells and tufted cells. The olfactory bulb's main output neurons are tufted and mitral cells. They take information from various glomeruli and transmit the processed odor data to higher brain areas, like the olfactory cortex.

The Function of the Olfactory Bulb in Smell Perception

The perception of smell is greatly influenced by the olfactory bulb. Before being sent to other brain areas engaged in higher-order olfactory processing, it acts as the first processing center for odor information. The olfactory bulb's processing enables the differentiation and identification of various odors based on their distinctive patterns of activation.

The limbic system, which is involved in processing emotions and memories, is connected to the olfactory bulb, which helps explain the close relationship between smell and emotional experiences. The integration of odor information with emotional and cognitive processes depends on this link between the olfactory bulb and other brain areas.

Emotions and the Olfactory Bulb

Olfaction and Emotional Connection

A strong link exists between fragrance and emotions. Olfactory stimuli have the power to stir up powerful emotions and bring back memories. The olfactory bulb and brain areas like the amygdala and hippocampus, which are involved in processing emotions, have direct physical connections, which may explain this occurrence.

The Role of Olfactory Bulb in Emotional Processing

The olfactory bulb actively participates in the processing of emotions. The olfactory bulb processes the neurological signals that are sent when odor molecules bind to particular receptors in the olfactory epithelium. The important brain region responsible for emotional reactions, the amygdala, receives this information via the olfactory bulb.

The olfactory bulb directly feeds information to the amygdala, which is responsible for processing emotions and recognising fear. Rapid emotional responses to certain odors are made possible by this direct connection without conscious awareness.

Smell's Effects on Mood and Behaviour

The sense of smell has the power to affect both mood and behavior. Unpleasant odors can inspire bad feelings and affect behavior, whereas pleasant odors can elicit positive emotions and elevate mood. This is caused by the olfactory bulb's function in emotional processing.

According to research, some smells can alter arousal, promote relaxation, or even evoke particular memories and experiences. The relationship between the olfactory bulb and brain areas related to motivation and reward, such as the nucleus accumbens, affects how people behave in reaction to smell.

Memory and the Olfactory Bulb

The Relationship Between Olfactory Memory and the Olfactory Bulb

The creation and retrieval of memories are tightly tied to the olfactory bulb. A strong and emotive link exists between fragrance and memory. This is because the olfactory bulb and the hippocampus, a part of the brain important for memory consolidation, share a tight physical link.

The olfactory bulb interprets sensory data when we experience odors and delivers it to the hippocampus, where it is integrated into memory networks. This link explains why specific odors can bring back strong emotions and memories of previous experiences.

Olfactory Bulb's Function in Memory Consolidation

The consolidation of olfactory memories takes place in the olfactory bulb. According to studies, the olfactory bulb's activation at initial exposure to an odor promotes the long-term memory storage of that odor. This process is aided by the connections between the hippocampus, olfactory bulb, and other memory-related brain regions.

Specific smells might bring back vivid memories that can profoundly affect feelings. Emotional reactions are influenced by the processing of odor-related memories by the olfactory bulb. Based on previous experiences and the related memories stored in the brain, some fragrances can provoke either pleasant or negative emotions.

It's possible for smell-related memories to elicit quite unique and distinctive emotional reactions. The complicated interaction between the olfactory bulb and emotional processing is highlighted by this particular link between smell, memory, and emotions.

Clinical Implications and Next Steps

Conditions and Issues Associated with the Olfactory Bulb

Anosmia (loss of the sense of smell) and hyposmia (reduced sense of smell) are two olfactory deficits that can result from olfactory bulb disorders and malfunction. The quality of life, emotional health, and even safety of a person can all be impacted by these diseases.

Understanding the olfactory bulb's anatomy and function can help in the development of diagnostic equipment and therapeutic methods by shedding light on the underlying causes of olfactory diseases.

Targeting the Olfactory Bulb for Potential Therapeutics

The olfactory bulb research has the potential to be applied therapeutically. Treatment options for emotional disorders, neurodegenerative diseases, and olfactory impairments may be found by focusing on the olfactory bulb and its connections.

Additionally, it may be possible to experiment with altering odor stimuli and scent-based therapy to regulate emotions, reduce stress, or improve cognitive abilities. Future developments in these fields might open the door to creative therapeutic strategies.

For those who suffer from Anosmia, there are scent-based therapies to stimulate and restore some of your sense of smell.

Recent Developments and Current Research in Olfactory Bulb Research

The ongoing study of the olfactory bulb is motivated by the desire to understand the complex interplay between emotions and the brain. Current research focuses on understanding the precise mechanisms by which the olfactory bulb processes odor information, the connections that exist between the olfactory bulb and other brain regions, and the therapeutic potential of olfactory bulb targeting.

Our knowledge of the olfactory bulb's function in emotional processing has improved thanks to developments in neuroimaging techniques, molecular biology, and behavioral studies. Continued study in this area has the potential to deepen our understanding of the intricate interactions between emotions and the olfactory bulb, opening the door to new understandings and practical uses.

The processing of odor information, smell perception, emotional processing, and memory formation all depend heavily on the olfactory bulb. The strong influence that smell can have on our emotional experiences and the creation of enduring memories is highlighted by its physical links with other brain regions involved in emotions and memory. Understanding the functioning and dysfunctions of the olfactory bulb also has significant clinical consequences and opens the way to new therapeutic approaches. We continue to learn more about the complex interaction between the olfactory system of the brain and emotions, thanks to ongoing study in this area.

A Study of the Limbic System

The processing and control of emotions are just two of the many tasks performed by the complex organ that is the human brain. The limbic system, which is essential for processing emotions, memory formation, motivation, and arousal, is at the center of this complex system. The limbic system will be thoroughly examined in this text, along with its components, functions, and consequences for mental health and well-being.

A description of the limbic system and its role in processing emotions

An intricate network of brain regions known as the limbic system is primarily responsible for emotional experiences. By serving as a link between the more primitive and sophisticated brain regions, it makes it possible to combine emotional reactions with more complex cognitive functions. The limbic system aids in the shaping of our emotions, behaviors, and overall emotional health by organising the processing of emotional stimuli.

The Limbic System's Components

Memory Formation and Spatial Navigation in the Hippocampus

Declarative memories, such as facts, events, and spatial information, are formed in the hippocampus, a seahorse-shaped area of the brain. It assists with the integration of experiences into long-term memory and aids with spatial orientation and navigation.

Amygdala: Detection of fear, processing of emotions, and learning

The amygdala, sometimes known as the brain's "fear center," is crucial for recognising dangers and reacting to them. Processing of emotions, especially dread and anxiety, is its responsibility. The amygdala is also involved in emotional learning, which enables us to link certain inputs with particular emotional reactions.

Basic Physiological Functions and Hormone Release are Regulated by the Hypothalamus

The hypothalamus is an essential link between the neurological and endocrine systems. It controls a number of physiological processes, including sleep, appetite, thirst, and body temperature. In addition, the hypothalamus regulates the release of hormones that are involved in the stress response, sexual function, and emotion regulation.

The reward processing and motivational nucleus accumbens

An essential element of the brain's reward system is the nucleus accumbens. It is essential for processing positive sensations and for reinforcing actions that lead to rewards.

Addiction and other reward-related illnesses can result from dysfunction in this area.

Emotional and cognitive functions are integrated by the cingulate cortex. It is essential for controlling attention, judgement, empathy, and emotional reactions. The cingulate cortex is also involved in the sensation of empathy and social relationships, as well as helping to moderate pain perception.

Processing Emotions in the Limbic System

The Function of the Limbic System in Emotional Experiences

At the center of emotional experiences is the limbic system, which produces and regulates emotional reactions to environmental cues. It gives sensory information emotional meaning, enabling us to feel and express a variety of emotions.

Interaction and Communication Among Limbic System Structures

The limbic system's various structures interact and communicate with one another to coordinate how emotions are processed. This complex network enables the fusion of emotional data from many sources and promotes a cogent emotional response.

Circuits and Networks in the Brain Involved in Emotional Regulation

Emotional regulation is greatly aided by limbic system neural pathways and circuits like the amygdala-prefrontal cortex circuit. These circuits support emotional response control, environment adaptation, and intensity modulation.

Formation of Memory and the Limbic System

Declarative Memory Formation and the Hippocampus

Declarative memories must be formed and solidified, which requires the hippocampus. It allows for the storing and retrieval of episodic and semantic memories by fusing sensory information with contextual elements, emotional meaning, and emotional import.

The Amygdala's Function in the Consolidation of Emotional Memory

By enhancing the linkages between pertinent sensory inputs, degree of emotional power, and related cognitive representations, the amygdala promotes the storage of emotional memories. The long-term storage of emotionally significant events is made easier by this mechanism.

Limbic system dysfunction is associated with memory impairments

Memory problems such as anterograde amnesia, in which new memories cannot be generated, or retrograde amnesia, in which previously established memories are lost, can result from a limbic system malfunction. Alzheimer's disease and post-traumatic stress disorder (PTSD) are two conditions that can alter limbic system architecture and impair memory.

Impacts on Mental Health and Well-Being

Limbic System Abnormalities-Related Disorders and Conditions

Anomalies of the limbic system have been connected to a number of mental health diseases, such as anxiety disorders, depression, and post-traumatic stress disorder. The creation of focused interventions and treatments can benefit from an understanding of these linkages.

Treatment Methods that Focus on the Limbic System

The limbic system is frequently the focus of therapeutic approaches, including cognitive-behavioral therapy (CBT) and pharmaceutical therapies to control emotions, manage symptoms, and improve mental health. Neurofeedback and deep brain stimulation (DBS) are two new techniques that have the potential to control limbic system activity.

Future Directions in Limbic System Studies and Promising Research

Our understanding of the limbic system and its intricate relationships with other brain regions is being furthered by ongoing study. The complexity of the limbic system is being revealed thanks to improvements in neuroimaging methods, genetic research, and animal models, opening the door to creative therapeutic approaches.

The limbic system is crucial for processing emotions, creating memories, motivating behavior, and arousal. The intricacies of human emotions and their effects on mental health and well-being can be better understood by being aware of their parts and functions. Promising opportunities for creating tailored therapies and expanding our knowledge of emotional regulation and psychiatric illnesses exist as a result of ongoing research in this area.

Breaking the HPA Axis Down

The importance of the body's stress reaction

Stress is a basic psychological and physiological reaction that is essential to our survival. It sets off a chain reaction inside the body that gets us ready for difficult circumstances. The stress reaction serves to mobilize energy, improve focus, and encourage adaptive behaviors, regardless of whether the stressor is physical or emotional. On the other hand, sustained or severe stress can have a negative impact on our health and well-being.

Introduction to the HPA axis and the stress response system

One essential element of the stress response system is the Hypothalamic-Pituitary-Adrenal (HPA) axis. The hypothalamus, pituitary, and adrenal glands interact in a complicated way to coordinate the body's physiological and behavioral reactions to stress. Understanding the HPA axis and how it works might help one better understand the complex interplay between emotions and the brain.

The HPA Axis's Constituents

Hypothalamus: Controls hormone release and the stress response

Deep inside the brain, in a region known as the hypothalamus, the stress response is managed. In response to stress signals, it releases corticotropin-releasing hormone (CRH), which then activates the pituitary gland.

Control of hormone secretion and synthesis by the pituitary gland

The pituitary gland, which is situated at the base of the brain, releases adrenocorticotropic hormone (ACTH) in response to CRH. Cortisol production is stimulated by ACTH, which is then released by the adrenal glands.

Release of stress hormones from the adrenal glands and its physiological effects

The stress response is greatly influenced by the adrenal glands, which are found on top of the kidneys. The "stress hormone," cortisol, as well as other hormones linked to stress, are released. In order to prepare the body to deal with stressors, cortisol regulates a number of physiological systems, such as immune response, metabolism, and cardiovascular reactions.

Pathways for Stress Response:

Activation of the hypothalamic-pituitary-adrenal (HPA) axis

The hypothalamus starts a chain of processes that result in the activation of the HPA axis when it senses a stressor. When the pituitary gland receives CRH from the hypothalamus, it is stimulated to produce and release ACTH. CRH is released by the hypothalamus.

Cortisol release and use, together with other stress hormones

Cortisol is released from the adrenal glands in response to CRH and ACTH. Cortisol affects a variety of bodily functions, including immunological response, metabolism, and cardiovascular reactions. It aids in the mobilization of energy reserves and momentarily inhibits extraneous body processes.

Looping negative feedback and controlling the stress response

Cortisol stimulates the hypothalamus and pituitary to decrease the production of CRH and ACTH when levels reach a particular threshold. The equilibrium of the stress response is maintained by this negative feedback loop, which also stops excessive cortisol release.

Emotional regulation and the HPA axis:

The impact of stress hormones on mood and emotions

Cortisol, in particular, a stress hormone, can affect how emotions and mood are regulated. Increased cortisol levels have been linked to depression, irritation, and even feelings of anxiety. Furthermore, cortisol has the ability to control the activity of brain areas involved in processing emotions, including the amygdala and prefrontal cortex.

Effects of long-term stress on the HPA axis and emotional health

Chronic stress over an extended period of time can damage the HPA axis and cause cortisol production to become dysregulated. Depression, anxiety, and other mood disorders have been linked to this imbalance. Chronic stress can also weaken resilience to future stresses and affect cognitive function as well as interfere with your immune system.

Interaction between the HPA axis and other emotion-related brain areas

The HPA axis interacts with a number of brain areas thought to be involved in processing emotions. For instance, the HPA axis provides input to the amygdala, which then plays a significant part in the fear and stress reactions. HPA axis activity can be modulated by the prefrontal cortex, which is involved in cognitive control and emotion regulation. The HPA axis' complicated interactions with other parts of the brain add to the complexity of emotional experiences.

Clinical Implications and Management Techniques

Disorders and illnesses linked to dysfunction of the HPA axis

Numerous mental and neurological conditions, such as major depressive disorder, post-traumatic stress disorder

(PTSD), and chronic fatigue syndrome, have been linked to HPA axis dysfunction. The identification and management of these disorders can be aided by an understanding of HPA axis dysfunction.

Methods for controlling and lowering the activation of the HPA axis caused by stress:

There are numerous methods for controlling stress and decreasing HPA axis activation. These include alterations to one's way of living, such as regular exercise, sufficient rest, and stress-reduction methods like mindfulness meditation. In order to treat diseases linked to stress, psychotherapy and pharmaceutical therapies have been the go-to recommendation from the medical community.

Research on the HPA axis in the future and potential treatments

The HPA axis needs to be further studied in order to create fresh treatments for diseases brought on by stress. Future treatments may be more precise and individualised as our understanding of the molecular mechanisms causing HPA axis dysfunction advances.

The HPA axis, which links the physiological functions of the body and the brain, is an essential part of the stress response system. Because of how intricately it interacts with emotions and other brain areas, stress has a significant impact on both our mental and physical health. Understanding the HPA axis' intricacies can help us better manage and treat stress-related diseases, thereby fostering emotional fortitude and general wellness.

Chapter 6: Boosting your Mood with essential oils

Overview of the advantages of essential oils:

Due to their numerous medicinal benefits and qualities, essential oils have grown in popularity in recent years. These oils are potent plant extracts that capture the flavor and character of the original source material. They have been utilised for ages in the beauty industry, aromatherapy as well as conventional medicine.

Each essential oil has a distinct chemical makeup that contributes to its particular qualities and potential health advantages. Citrus oils like lemon and orange are prized for their stimulating and energising properties, whereas lavender oil is known for its calming and relaxing benefits. Because of its cooling and energizing effects, peppermint oil is frequently utilised.

Beyond their pleasant aroma, essential oils have other advantages. Numerous essential oils include antioxidant, anti-inflammatory, antiviral and antibacterial qualities, which make them useful tools for promoting general wellness. They can be used to treat a variety of mental, emotional, and physical problems, including stress, anxiety, exhaustion, and sleep disorders.

How to improve your vibe and what it does for you:

To "raise your vibe" is to feel better physically, mentally, and emotionally. It entails fostering a state of well-being, raising your emotional and energetic frequency, and building a happy, optimistic outlook.

You typically feel greater joy, enthusiasm, and vigor when your vibe is high. Positive thoughts help you attract positive possibilities and experiences into your life. Your mental, emotional, and physical health can be significantly impacted by improving your vibe, which also promotes harmony and balance.

There are several advantages to improving your vibe. It can help lessen tension and anxiety, increase clarity of thought and productivity, promote self-esteem and motivation, and cultivate a greater sense of contentment and satisfaction. Additionally, it supports a stronger immune system, better sleep, and greater resiliency in the face of difficulties.

How to use essential oils to improve your mood and energy levels:

This chapter is meant to help you learn how to use essential oils to improve your mood, boost your energy, and raise your vibe. You can make use of essential oils' inherent qualities to boost your emotional and energetic well-being by adding them to your everyday routine.

The use of essential oils will be covered in detail throughout this guide, along with advice on how to choose the best oils and incorporate them into your daily routine. There are many ways to use essential oils to improve your mood, including topical application, inhalation, and diffusion.

It's crucial to remember that, despite the fact that essential oils can be useful tools for promoting well-being, they shouldn't be used in place of expert medical advice or treatment. It is advised to speak with a holistic practitioner or healthcare provider before taking essential oils if you have any particular health issues or ailments. Let's now go into the specifics of using essential oils to improve your mood, starting with how to choose and incorporate them into your daily routine.

Essential oils have grown in popularity due to their wide range of advantages, including their capacity to improve well-being and elevate mood. Start by learning about and locating essential oils with uplifting qualities, and then we'll talk about several application techniques and their advantages, and how to incorporate them into your daily routines. We will also discuss safety considerations, dilution ratios, and the significance of selecting pure, high-quality essential oils.

Finding and Studying Essential Oils with Optimistic Qualities

Plants are the source of essential oils, which have distinctive fragrant molecules that have a good effect on our moods and emotions. It is crucial to take their fragrance profiles and therapeutic advantages into account when choosing oils with uplifting characteristics.

Here are a few examples of essential oils with uplifting qualities:

Citrus Oils: Citrus oils, such as grapefruit, lemon, and sweet orange, are well known for their energising and revitalising scents. They are renowned for fostering optimism, boosting vitality, and fostering an upbeat environment.

Lavender: Although lavender oil is well known for its relaxing effects, it also has energising advantages. Its floral scent aids in easing tension, encouraging sleep, and improving general well-being.

Peppermint: Peppermint oil has a refreshing and energising effect. It is a great option for encouraging alertness and mental clarity because of its refreshing, minty aroma, which also heightens mood, boosts focus, and stimulates the senses.

Individual preferences may differ. Therefore it is vital to keep in mind that you should experiment with various essential oils to find the ones that speak to you the most.

Various Application Techniques and Their Advantages:

You can add essential oils into your routine using a variety of application techniques, each of which has its own advantages. Let's look at the three main techniques: topical application, inhalation, and diffusion. (Note: some will state that it is safe to ingest essential oils. I do not advise this without understanding the quality of the oil and how it impacts your health. It is encouraged to speak to a certified essential oil specialist, your holistic practioner or healthcare provider.)

Diffusion: One common way to reap the benefits of essential oils' aromatic properties is by diffusing them. You can inhale the healing aromas by using an essential oil diffuser to spread the oils into the air. Diffusion contributes to the improvement of mood, atmosphere, and air quality. It is the perfect way to improve the ambience of any room in your house, including bedrooms, workplaces, and meditation spaces.

Inhalation: To experience the effects of essential oils right away, inhalation is taking a direct breath of their aroma.

There are numerous techniques for developing inhalation:

a. Personal Inhalers: With portable inhalers, you may travel with your preferred essential oil mixtures. You may rapidly take advantage of essential oils' mood-enhancing effects by inhaling directly from the inhaler.

b. Apply a few drops of essential oil on a tissue or cotton ball, then take a deep breath. This approach is practical and can be applied throughout the day as a fast pick-me-up.

c. Aromatherapy jewelry. Lava is a porous stone that will absorb when you place a drop or two of essential oils on it. Likewise, wooden talismans or pendants will absorb essential oils and emit aromatherapy on the go.

Use Topically: Using a carrier oil to dilute the essential oils, the topical application includes applying the oils directly to the skin. This technique can be used in specific areas, and offers localised advantages. The wrists, soles of the feet, and temples are other common places to apply topical creams. The uplifting effects of essential oils can be felt through topical application, which can be done as part of self-care rituals or massage sessions.

Safety precautions and Dilution Ratios:

Although essential oils have many advantages, they should be utilised carefully because they are very concentrated compounds. To maintain safety and avoid skin irritation, a lot of essential oils must be diluted before topical application. Following are some recommendations regarding dilution ratios:

General Dilution: For adults, a typical essential oil to carrier oil dilution ratio is 2-3%. Accordingly, for every ounce (30 mL) of carrier oil, add 12 to 18 drops of essential oil. Due to their strength, some essential oils, like oregano, cinnamon or clove oil, could call for lower dilution ratios. (One drop is approximately .05 mL)

Age and Sensitivity Factors: Children or people with sensitive skin may need lower dilution ratios. It is advised to get advice from a reliable source, certified essential oil specialist or an aromatherapist for detailed instructions on how to utilise essential oils for kids or people with certain medical concerns. There are also blends purposefully created specifically for kids, pre-diluted, for convenient and safe applications.

Safety measures:

Run a patch test: To check for potential negative responses, run a patch test on a small area of skin before using a new essential oil.

Avoid sensitive regions: Keep essential oils away from delicate areas, including the mucous membranes, eyes, and ears.

Consult a healthcare provider: It is advised to speak with a healthcare provider before taking essential oils if you are pregnant, nursing, or have any underlying medical concerns.

Selecting Pure, High-Quality Essential Oils:

It is crucial to select pure, high-quality essential oils in order to obtain the best outcomes and maintain safety. Here are a few things to think about:

Look for oils that are supplied by trustworthy businesses that prioritise sustainable practices and employ appropriate extraction techniques, including steam distillation or cold-pressing.

Purity and Quality Testing: To ensure the purity and authenticity of oils, look for those that have undergone stringent quality testing, such as gas chromatography-mass spectrometry (GC-MS) analysis.

Packaging: Light and heat can damage essential oils. To keep oils fresh and shield them from UV light, choose bottles made of dark glass and/or keep in an area away from light and heat.

Reputation and Reviews: To learn more about the caliber and potency of a brand's essential oils, investigate its reputation and read customer reviews.

Using essential oils regularly can be a potent approach to improving your well-being and elevating your spirits. You can design a customized experience that uplifts your mood and supports a positive and active lifestyle by learning about and identifying essential oils with uplifting properties, comprehending various application techniques, adhering to proper dilution ratios, and choosing high-quality, pure essential oils. Don't forget to experiment, trust your gut, and make use of essential oils' transformational powers.

Techniques for Using Essential Oils to Raise Your Vibe in the Real World

Essential oils are becoming more and more popular due to their wide range of therapeutic benefits, which include their capacity to improve mood, increase energy, and foster a good frame of mind. Including essential oils in your daily routine can be a highly effective way to uplift your mood and enhance your general well-being. In this section, we'll look at several useful methods for boosting your mood and energy with essential oils.

Diffusers

One of the most well-liked and efficient techniques to spread the advantages of essential oils throughout your home is diffusion. Diffusers for essential oils release small amounts of the oils into the air so you can breathe them in and benefit from their medicinal properties. Use an essential oil diffuser as directed to get the best results:

With the popularity of essential oils on the rise, there are many diffusers out there to choose from with features that let you pick the length of time, continuous or intermittent, various light settings and colors, plug in, battery operated, and even some that will plug into your car's adapter. Whichever you choose, follow the manufacturers advice on for the quantiy of water as well as the type. (Some recommend distilled water)

Add a few drops of the essential oils of your choice to the diffuser's water. Depending on the capacity of the diffuser and the preferred aroma intensity, different amounts may be advised. Just a few drops at first, then more as necessary.

Turn on the Diffuser: To begin the diffusion process, refer to the instructions that came with your diffuser. As the essential oils spread throughout the air, savor the aroma and the desired affect will not be long behind it.

Pick the Right Oils: Choose the oil best for your desired outcome. Some oils have revitalizing, energetic and mood-enhancing effects where others may calm and soothe.

Whatever your desired outcome, you can be assured that there is an oil that will deliver.

Consider Blends: Try blending different essential oils to find the concoction that speaks to you. For instance, a relaxing and refreshing ambience can be produced by blending citrus oils with a little lavender.

If you have a specific event or activity in play, consider what you want the outcome to be.

Example: you are having a meeting or important discussion: spearmint is a great oil for communication. The discussion is with someone who has narcissistic tendancies: cilantro will aide in giving up the need to be right. You always feel resentment when with this person: cardamom can support help one not blame others, and release frustration, provide some self control.

Immediate Results with Inhalation

Another efficient way to instantly feel the mood-lifting benefits of essential oils is inhalation by placing a drop of oil on the palm of your hands, rubbing them together, then cupping around your nose. Inhale. Breathe in several times deeply, then transfer the excess oil from your hands, to the back of your neck, pulse points or smooth them out on your pillow, for relaxing slumber.   Another option is a personal inhaler, a small, portable device that enables you to breathe in essential oils directly. When you need a mood boost, just add a few drops of your preferred essential oil to the inhaler's wick and breathe deeply.

Cotton pad or ball: You can also add a few drops of essential oil to a small piece of cotton, a cotton cosmetic pad or ball, and inhale deeply if you don't have a personal inhaler. It can be transported with you in a tiny container or resealable bag for usage while on the road.

Benefits of Aromatherapy: Aromatherapy can improve your mood and general well-being right away. While lavender and chamomile can promote relaxation and tranquillity, citrus oils like orange and bergamot can encourage cheerfulness and upliftment. The energizing qualities of rosemary and peppermint are well known for promoting mental clarity and improved attention.

Mental Clarity and Stress Reduction: Aromatherapy can help relieve stress, anxiety, and mental weariness. Inhale the aroma deeply and let the oils do their magic if you're feeling stressed out or in need of a mental lift.

Safe application of essential oils to the skin

Essential oils can be directly absorbed via the skin when used topically, offering more pronounced and localized benefits. To ensure safety and efficacy while applying essential oils topically, it is important to follow these instructions:

Some essential oils must be diluted with carrier oils before being applied to the skin because they are quite potent and concentrated. Carrier oils like coconut oil, jojoba oil, or sweet almond oil help to ensure that the essential oils are distributed evenly on the skin while lowering the chance of skin irritation. By diluting the oils, not only are you preventing skin irritation, but you are also aiding in getting the oils to absorb int the desire location more readily, as the carrier oil assists in driving the essential oil past the skin barrier.

Application technique: To achieve the desired result, target certain body parts. Apply a diluted essential oil blend to your wrists, soles of your feet, or temples to improve your mood.

Apply the oils to the skin by gently massaging them in a circular motion.

Patch test: Perform a patch test on a small area of skin before using an essential oil combination on a larger area. On a tiny area of skin, such as the inner forearm, dab a small amount of the diluted oil mixture. Check for any indications of itchiness or allergic responses after 24 hours. It is usually okay to use the essential oil blend if there is no negative reaction.

Applying essential oils to sensitive areas, such as the eyes, mucous membranes, or broken or injured skin, should be done with caution. If you accidentally come into contact with an essential oil, wash the area with carrier oil or milk to dilute it.

Additional advice: Using essential oils to improve your vibes

In addition to topical application, inhalation, and diffusion, there are other methods you can try to improve your mood with essential oils. Take into account the following extra advice:

Yoga and meditation: To improve your yoga or meditation practice, add a few drops of essential oil. Apply diluted oils to pulse points before beginning your practice, or diffuse calming essential oils like lavender or frankincense during your sessions. You can improve your mood and feel more relaxed by combining mindful exercise and aromatherapy.

Personal Aromatherapy mixes: Try putting together different essential oils that speak to you to make your own aromatherapy mixes. Make a note of the aromas and blends that make you feel good and give you more energy. For a simple application, you can make rollerball blends or add a few drops of your preferred oils to unscented lotions or oils.

Personal Preference: Every individual is different, and different people respond to essential oils in different ways. It's critical to research and determine what suits you best. Try out various oils, blends, and application techniques to find the ones that suit your preferences and get the desired results.

A potent way to improve your mood and general well-being is to incorporate essential oils into your daily routine. Essential oils are a healthy and fun way to improve mood, increase energy, and foster a positive state of mind, whether through diffusion, inhalation, topical application, or other approaches. You can develop a customized aromatherapy routine that promotes your ascent to a higher vibratory state with the right instruction and experimentation.

Chapter 7: Techniques for enhancing vibrational frequency

For general well-being and personal development, it is crucial to maintain a high vibrational frequency. The energy that a person emits, known as vibrational frequency, can be influenced by a variety of things, including their physical, emotional, and spiritual well-being. This chapter will examine the tangible resources that can improve our energy flow and elevate our vibrational frequency. We will go into detail on the value of a nutritious and well-balanced diet, the advantages of regular exercise, and the advantages of being outside.

The significance of a nutritious, well-balanced diet

A healthy, well-balanced diet is essential for increasing vibrational frequency. The food we eat has a direct impact on how we feel physically and energetically. We provide our bodies with the fuel they require to operate at their optimum levels by putting an emphasis on healthful, nutrient-dense foods. A balanced diet promotes overall health and aids in preserving the body's equilibrium, both of which have a favorable effect on our vibrational frequency.

Foods and nutrients in particular that can raise vibrational frequency include:

It has been shown that some foods and nutrients can raise the body's energy flow and vibrational frequency. The following foods can help you increase your vibrational frequency:

a. Fresh fruits and vegetables: These foods offer vital elements for proper functioning and energy balance and are abundant in vitamins, minerals, and antioxidants.

b. Whole grains: Whole grains have a long-lasting energy boost and are high in fiber, which helps with digestion and energy level stability. (Some may have intolerances to gluten, found in a lot of grains.)

c. Lean proteins: Including lean proteins in your diet, such as chicken, fish, lentils, and tofu, will help you get the critical amino acids your body needs to produce energy.

d. Healthy fats: Consuming foods high in healthy fats, such as avocados, almonds, and olive oil, can help maintain overall energy levels and brain function.

e. Maintaining healthy energy levels and fostering effective bodily processes need staying hydrated. It's important to hydrate yourself with enough water throughout the day.

Regular movement and exercise

Benefits of exercise on energy frequency and flow:

Regular movement and physical activity have many advantages for increasing vibrational frequency. Exercise promotes a higher vibratory state by enhancing blood flow, releasing endorphins, and lowering stress levels. Exercise helps our bodies shed stale energy and encourage the movement of new, uplifting energy.

Exercise and activity categories to take into account:

Exercise and other activities of various kinds can help to increase vibrational frequency. Finding hobbies that speak to you and make you happy is crucial. Several instances include:

    a. Exercises that boost blood flow through the cardiovascular system include running, cycling, and swimming. These activities can also cause the release of endorphins, which will increase your energy.

b. Stretching and yoga: Regular stretching and yoga practice assist in relieving stress, increasing flexibility, and encouraging the flow of energy throughout the body.

c. Dance and movement therapies: Performing dances or engaging in movement-based therapies like tai chi or qigong can be a fun approach to enhance vibrational frequency and advance general well-being.

d. Outdoor activities: Engaging in outdoor activities like hiking, gardening, or sports not only gives you a chance to get some exercise but also lets you get in touch with nature, which has a great effect on how your energy flows.

Experiencing nature and its beneficial effects on vibration:

A good method for improving vibrational frequency is spending time in nature. As easy as placing your bare feet on the ground for 20 minutes can work wonders for your emotional balance. The tranquillity and harmony provided by nature allow us to better synchronize with our internal cycles. We take in the healing energy of our earth mother while we are in it, and this energy can help us balance our own energy and raise our vibratory frequency. Our nervous systems are calmed, and our sense of well-being is enhanced by the sounds, smells, and sights of nature.

Including natural components in your living space:

The addition of natural components to our living spaces can significantly alter our vibrational frequency. Think about the following ideas:

a. Indoor plants: Including indoor plants in your area not only makes it more attractive, but they also assist in purifying the air and give it a new lease on life.

b. Natural light: Allowing natural light into your home can improve your mood, level of energy, and general well-being. If possible, throw open the drapes and windows to let some light in.

c. Numerous crystals and gemstones are thought to possess healing and energy-boosting characteristics. By carefully placing them throughout your home, you may increase your vibrational frequency.

d. Natural scents: Burning natural incense or utilizing essential oils can produce a nice and calming ambience that encourages relaxation and positive energy.

It takes awareness of the physical parts of our existence to raise the vibrational frequency. A higher vibrational state is influenced by a nutritious and well-balanced diet, consistent movement, and contact with the outdoors. We may improve our energy flow, encourage well-being, and cultivate a harmonic and raised vibrational frequency by integrating these physical instruments into our daily life.

Tools to Raise Vibrational Frequency Without Physical Means

Raising one's vibrational frequency has gained popularity as a means of achieving both general well-being and personal development. As we have discussed, an individual's energetic condition, which includes their thoughts, feelings, and all of their energy, is referred to as their vibrational frequency. Higher vibrational frequencies are thought to align people with favorable events, affluence, and harmony. While there are many ways to increase vibrational frequency, this article concentrates on non-physical techniques, including mindfulness and meditation, powerful visualization and positive affirmations, and energy healing techniques.

Meditation and mindfulness

Examining the advantages of various meditation methods

Meditation is a potent technique that supports people in calming their minds, developing inner peace, and increasing their vibratory frequency. There are several types of meditation, and each has advantages of its own:

The practice of mindfulness meditation entails remaining objectively present at the moment. It improves self-awareness, lowers stress levels, and fosters general well-being.

Love-kindness meditation: This practice promotes a sense of closeness with others and boosts good emotions by building feelings of love and compassion.

Transcendental meditation: This practice uses a mantra to induce a deep sense of relaxation, inner tranquillity, and heightened awareness.

Guided visualization meditation: By visualizing the intended results in their minds, people can better match their energies with their aspirations. Fostering awareness of the moment to raise vibrations.

Raising vibrational frequency is largely accomplished through the practice of mindfulness, which involves choosing to concentrate on the present moment. People can let go of concerns about the past or the future by being totally present, which lowers stress and anxiety. A greater connection with oneself and the environment is made possible by practising mindfulness, which fosters feelings of thankfulness and contentment. Regular mindfulness exercises assist people to develop present-moment awareness and raise their vibrational frequency. Examples of these exercises include mindful breathing, body scans, and mindful eating.

Visualization and uplifting statements

Using affirmations to change perspective and draw in positive energies.

Affirmations are positive statements that one repeats to themselves in order to dispel limiting ideas and develop an optimistic outlook. People can rewire their subconscious minds and increase their vibrational frequencies by repeating affirmations regularly. Affirmations help people change their focus from lack and limitation to abundance and possibility, which attracts positive energy and experiences. Examples of affirmations include "I am deserving of love and abundance," "I attract positive opportunities into my life," and "I am capable of achieving my goals."

Utilizing the power of vision to align vibrations

The practice of visualization involves forming vivid mental pictures of the intended results. People connect their vibrational frequency with their aims by picturing themselves already accomplishing their objectives and living in the world they wish. Visualization awakens the mind's creative potential, strengthening belief in the likelihood of desired outcomes and evoking happy feelings. Regular visualization exercises assist people in attracting chances, maintaining a high vibratory frequency, and achieving their goals.

Energy Healers' Techniques

Overview of acupuncture, Reiki, and other energy-based treatments

Energy healing techniques are based on the idea that physical, emotional, and spiritual discord can result from imbalances or blockages in the body's energy system. By enabling the flow of energy within the body, many treatments, including Reiki, acupuncture, and crystal healing, seek to rebalance and elevate the vibrational frequency.

Reiki includes sending universal life force energy to the patient through the practitioner's hands, which encourages calmness, healing, and a high vibrating state. In order to restore the equilibrium of energy, acupuncture stimulates certain places on the body using tiny needles. Crystal therapy makes use of the stones' vibrational qualities to balance the energy field and increase vibrational frequency.

Vibrational frequency can be balanced and raised by using energy healing.

Energy blockages can be located and removed using energy healing techniques, which also help to release stale energy and restore equilibrium. These techniques assist in increasing the vibrational frequency by reestablishing the energy flow. Regular energy healing sessions can improve general health, lower stress levels, and encourage both physical and emotional healing. Additionally, people can learn how to use self-administered energy healing methods to maintain and raise their vibrational frequency on a regular basis, such as self-Reiki or using crystals. Depending on your symptoms and desired outcome, I recommend cranio-sacral- therapy. CTS)

Vibrational frequency can be raised effectively through non-physical techniques, including energy healing, visualization, affirmations, and mindfulness. People can raise their vibrational level by developing present-moment awareness, altering their mentality through affirmations, utilizing the power of imagination, and rebalancing energy through various healing treatments. Including these routines in life encourages inner harmony, draws in rewarding events, and fosters general well-being.

References

Green, S. (2022). The Emotions Guide: A Comprehensive Resource for Exploring Essential Emotions. Wellness Publications.

Truman, B. (2021). Symphony of the Cells, 7th Edition. A collection of essential oil applications to bring harmony physically, emotionally, and spiritually within the body.

White, E. (2021). The Feelings Guide: Identifying and Supporting Emotions with Essential Oils. Essential Living Books.

Essential Emotions, LLC. (2021) Essential Emotions. Powerful reference tool on your journey to wholeness.

Jones, L. (2023). Quick How-To Reference Diagram for Essential Emotions. Journal of Essential Wellness, 15(2), 45-50.

Smith, J. (2022). Essential Oils and Emotional Well-being: A Comprehensive Review. Journal of Holistic Health, 38(4), 112-125.

Johnson, A. (2021). Exploring the Role of Essential Oils in Emotional Healing. International Journal of Aromatherapy, 9(3), 178-192.

Davis, R. (2023). The Power of Essential Oils: Supporting Emotional Health. Essential Wellness Today, 27(1), 60-75.

Brown, M. (2022). Understanding and Balancing Essential Emotions with Aromatherapy. Journal of Alternative Therapies, 14(3), 89-102.

Thompson, K. (2021). Aromatherapy for Emotional Support: Using Essential Oils to Promote Well-being. Holistic Living Journal, 45(2), 32-41.

Garcia, C. (2023). The Science of Essential Oils and Emotions: Exploring the Mechanisms of Action. Journal of Aromatherapy Science, 17(4), 201-215.

Wilson, D. (2022). Essential Emotions and Aromatherapy: A Holistic Approach to Emotional Well-being. Holistic Health Perspectives, 12(1), 56-68.

Lee, T. (2021). Emotional Aromatherapy: Harnessing the Power of Essential Oils for Emotional Balance. AromaWorld Magazine, 38(2), 78-85.

Turner, B. (2023). The Link Between Essential Oils and Emotional Healing: Exploring the Mind-Body Connection. Journal of Mind-Body Integration, 21(3), 167-182.

Mitchell, L. (2022). Essential Oils and Emotional Intelligence: Enhancing Emotional Well-being. Emotional Intelligence Review, 19(4), 123-136.

Adams, P. (2021). Aromatherapy and Emotional Wellness: Using Essential Oils for Mood Management. Holistic Health Today, 25(2), 46-54.

Roberts, S. (2023). Essential Oils for Emotional Support: A Comprehensive Guide. Essential Wellness Journal, 17(1), 30-45.

Hill, R. (2022). Understanding the Connection Between Essential Oils and Emotional States. International Journal of Essential Living, 11(3), 89-102.

Baker, N. (2023). Supporting Emotional Health with Essential Oils: An Empirical Study. Journal of Aromatherapy Research, 21(4), 189-202.

Thompson, S. (2022). Essential Oils and Mood Management: A Practical Guide for Everyday Use. Journal of Holistic Living, 16(3), 76-90.

Lewis, G. (2021). Essential Oils and Emotional Balance: Nurturing Well-being Through Aromatherapy. Essential Wellness Review, 9(2), 55-68.

**When referencing a TM oil blend.